D1417907

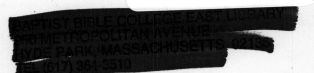

READING DISABILITY:
Progress and Research Needs in Dyslexia

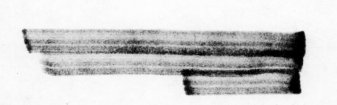

READING DISABILITY

PROGRESS AND RESEARCH NEEDS IN DYSLEXIA

edited by John Money

Baltimore
The Johns Hopkins Press
1962

© 1962 by The Johns Hopkins Press, Baltimore 18, Md.

Distributed in Great Britain by Oxford University Press, London

Printed in the United States of America

Library of Congress Catalog Card Number: 62-14360

Second Printing, 1963

Third Printing, 1964

Preface

The Johns Hopkins Conference on Research Needs and Prospects in Dyslexia and Related Aphasic Disorders was convened at the Johns Hopkins Medical Institutions on November 15-17, 1961, under the auspices of the departments of Pediatrics, Psychiatry and Ophthalmology, and received the unqualified endorsement of the heads of these three departments, Professors Robert E. Cooke, Seymour S. Kety, and A. Edward Maumenee, respectively.

The conference owed its inception to the interest of Herman Krieger Goldberg, M.D., Assistant Professor of Ophthalmology, in the practicing ophthalmologist's problems and responsibilities with regard to children who, referred because of severe handicap in learning to read, nonetheless have normal, healthy vision. Dr. Goldberg was host to the participants and other guests at the conference's opening reception and dinner meeting.

That there was a conference at all is due to the generosity of the Association for the Aid of Crippled Children, which underwrote the entire expense.

The size of the conference was restricted to that of a small seminar with 13 participants and an average of a dozen auditors. The participants prepared their papers beforehand and a copy of every paper was supplied to each participant and auditor in advance. In the conference room, speakers gave a brief exposition of their papers, a greater amount of time being reserved for discussions. The proceedings were tape recorded, with excellent results, for reference and filing. In addition, Mrs. Beverly Schmidt took extensive shorthand notes and Dr. C. Keith Conners made extensive synoptic notes during the conference to supplement my own. It was from the beginning planned not to publish the verbatim discussions, but to prepare instead a synoptic postconference review which would incorporate the main themes emergent from the discussion (Chapter 1). The papers themselves are published substantially unchanged.

I wish to put on record the excellence of the secretarial and editorial assistance of Mrs. Beverly Schmidt in processing the manuscripts for the press.

JOHN MONEY

Conference Faculty

Convener

John Money, Ph.D.   Associate Professor of Medical Psychology and Pediatrics, The Johns Hopkins University, Baltimore 5, Maryland.

Chairman of Sessions

Leon Eisenberg, M.D.   Professor of Child Psychiatry, The Johns Hopkins University, Baltimore 5, Maryland.

Participants

Arthur L. Benton, Ph.D.   Professor of Psychology and Neurology, State University of Iowa, Iowa City, Iowa.

Norman Geschwind, M.D.   Chief, Aphasia Unit, Section of Neurology, Boston Veterans Administration Hospital, Boston Massachusetts; and Research Associate, Section of Psychology, Massachusetts Institute of Technology, Cambridge 39, Massachusetts.

William G. Hardy, Ph.D.   Associate Professor of Otolaryngology and of Environmental Medicine; and Director, Hearing and Speech Clinic, The Johns Hopkins Medical Institutions, Baltimore 5, Maryland.

Davis Howes, Ph.D. Associate Professor of Psychology, Massachusetts Institute of Technology, Cambridge 39, Massachusetts; and Consultant in Neuropsychology, Boston Veterans Administration Hospital, Boston, Massachusetts.

John R. Newbrough, Ph.D. Project Director, Community Projects Section, Mental Health Study Center, Program Development, Institute of Mental Health, Silver Spring, Maryland.

Heinz F. R. Prechtl, Ph.D. Chief, Department of Experimental Neurology, University of Groningen, The Netherlands.

Ralph D. Rabinovitch, M.D. Director, The Hawthorn Center, Northville, Michigan.

Roger E. Saunders, M.A. Psychologist, Board of Education of Baltimore County, Towson 4, Maryland.

Gilbert Schiffman, Ed.M., O.D. Supervisor, Corrective-Remedial Reading, Board of Education of Baltimore County, Towson 4, Maryland; Professorial Lecturer, Loyola College; and Assistant in Medical Psychology, The Johns Hopkins University, Baltimore, Maryland.

Joseph M. Wepman, Ph.D. Professor of Psychology and Surgery, The University of Chicago, Chicago 37, Illinois.

Oliver L. Zangwill, M.A. Professor of Experimental Psychology, The Psychological Laboratory, Cambridge University, Cambridge, England.

Participants in Absentia

Herbert G. Birch, Ph.D., M.D. Associate Research Professor, Department of Pediatrics, Albert Einstein College of Medicine, New York 61, New York.

James G. Kelly, Ph.D., S.M.Hyg. Chief, Community Projects Section, Mental Health Study Center, Program Development, Institute of Mental Health, Silver Spring, Maryland.

Contents

READING DISABILITY:

Progress and Research Needs in Dyslexia

Introduction

LEON EISENBERG

It is altogether appropriate that a conference on the topic of reading disability should be convened under the auspices of the Association for the Aid of Crippled Children. A handicap in reading is a crippling disorder in a society that is increasingly dependent upon literacy. When the avenue to printed material is blocked, the individual not only has the treasures of literature forever closed to him, but he will also find increasing difficulty in earning a living, finding his way about in our complex cities, and assimilating the information necessary for an adequate social adjustment. Those corners of society in which a nonreader might secret himself and be undistinguishable from his literate contemporaries are well nigh nonexistent.

It is a matter of considerable importance to be aware of the different senses in which the concept of reading disability is employed. For, as I think all will agree, any hope of discriminating causes and providing treatment will depend upon the differentiation of one type of disorder from another. To begin with, there are those who cannot read as the result of a sensory handicap, as

3

in the case of extremely poor vision or hearing. Next there are those whose inability to read is part of a general pattern of inability to learn, namely the mentally deficient. The third group is made up of those children who have had deficient or improper instruction by virtue of insufficient or poor schooling. A fourth group can be said to be made up of those children who, despite an educational opportunity, are so poorly motivated to learn to read because of circumstances at home that they continue to lag behind their grade norms. It is my view that for none of these groups would the term, "specific dyslexia," be appropriate. For I would apply this term to a situation in which a child is unable to learn to read with proper facility despite normal intelligence, intact senses, proper instruction, and normal motivation. It is evident that in this construction the term "specific" really implies an idiopathic condition, that is, one whose cause is unknown.

If one were to do a large-scale survey in order to determine reading levels among school children, one's net would catch a large number of children reading below their grade levels, of whom I would guess a minority would be children with specific dyslexia. But if this entire group were to be treated as though it were made up of homogeneous cases, the investigator would almost certainly not come to valid conclusions about causes or effective treatments because one class would not be distinguished from another. I suspect that one could discriminate among the groups a posteriori by measuring their responses to remedial programs. Those with sensory handicaps would acquire reading facility once the sensory deficit was recognized and corrected. Those suffering from inadequate instruction would profit once better teaching was provided. If one had methods to motivate the unmotivated, by definition there would be a change in reading level. But among the failures would remain the mentally defective and the specifically dyslexic. These two in turn could be discriminated on the basis of their responses to a general program of education, since the dyslexic is often quite successful in other studies so long as they are not primarily dependent upon his reading skill.

From everything we know about children, we would expect that success in a program of remedial reading would be the greater, the earlier the child's deficits were detected and corrective measures instituted. (Unfortunately, we still lack specific methods of distinguishing the true dyslexic from the child who is slow or late in learning to read but who will learn while still within the primary grades) Since our public-school system is overcrowded and remedial reading is costly and often unavailable, it has become customary to delay the institution of corrective programs until the third grade or later when the true dyslexic will have segregated himself from the "late bloomer." This undoubtedly effects an economy from the standpoint of the administrator in that special instructions are not needlessly provided for children who are in any event going to learn. But this economizing is accomplished at a heavy cost to the dyslexic child. For by the time the remedial program is offered to him, he has had several years of failure, with a consequent development of aversion to reading and related activities, as well as of emotional problems related to feelings of inadequacy. Whether or not there may be an additional deficit related to faulty learning or even deviant maturation we do not at this point know. But I would argue in favor of providing extra help and special instruction even for those not actually in need of them in order to be certain that optimal help is provided to those who certainly require it. It is evident that, once we have specific methods of diagnosis that are reliable and are applicable in the field, this indiscriminate process of special tutoring will no longer be necessary.

There are many who hold that specific reading disability is in large part an emotional disorder. They argue for this thesis on the basis of clinical observations of dyslexic children who for the most part show definite evidence of such disorder. But it should be clear that emotional disorder is almost inevitably a consequence of the repeated frustration entailed in trying, but being unable, to learn to read. The disentangling of causes and effect once the problem is well set is quite complex, if not impossible. Again, an a posteriori judgment may sometimes be made with confidence on the basis of the response to specific corrective measures. In the experience of most clinicians, the child whose reading deficit is secondary to an emotional problem is likely to show a rather rapid gain in reading skills once an effective treatment for the emotional disorder has been introduced. I would add only that in my experience even such children seem to require remedial reading instruction before they can make up for their deficit, though the rapidity of their response distinguishes them sharply from children with a specific dyslexia. Among the latter, remedial reading is most often a painfully slow process with small gains despite large efforts, and, at times there is unfortunately no visible gain at all. I distinguish in this discussion between the child with poor motivation (which I take to be the result of social class orientation and family attitudes toward learning) and the one with emotional disturbance. In a sense, however, both categories may be quite similar since one can explain the reading disability secondary to emotional disorder in terms of a poor motivation for learning.

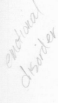

The task of evaluating the effectiveness of proposed programs for remedial reading is no less difficult than the one of separating etiological groups. For if a child fails to improve after a program of reading retraining, he is said to be unresponsive to remedial reading techniques. But it should be obvious that there is a wide variety of remedial reading techniques; each of them depends not only on the theoretical premises of the system but as well upon the particular skills, personality, and attitudes of the remedial reading teacher. Teaching by any method requires that there be a relationship between teacher and pupil; and a good remedial reading teacher often not only assists the child in his reading problem but is helpful to him in establishing a more successful adjustment in other ways as well. The teacher who may be familiar with the proper technical method but does not succeed in gaining the confidence and the attention of her pupil is likely to fail. Thus, if we are asked to evaluate the results of remedial reading instruction, we must in turn ask: What methods are applied by what teacher to what category of cases?

These few clinical remarks may serve to introduce a symposium which has been rather deliberately pitched at the level of basic investigation rather than clinical case discussion or field method. In this approach, it is necessary that we challenge the most elementary assumptions and question the validity of currently available methods. I beg the indulgence of the clinician toward the skeptical attitude of the investigators. It is not that there is no appreciation of the complexities of the problem the clinician must face nor the devotion and effort he applies to his task, but that nothing must be taken for granted if we are to arrive at any fundamental understanding of the basic problems involved. At the outset of this conference, I dare say we all agree that we do not expect to have the answers by its end. We can hope at least that we will have discovered some of the questions we must ask.

1

Dyslexia: A Postconference Review*

JOHN MONEY

Differential Classification

Dyslexia means defective reading. The reading defect may represent loss of competency following brain injury or degeneration; or it may represent a developmental failure to profit from reading instruction.

Technically, it is correct to say that an unschooled aboriginal of some primitive tribe is alexic or, if educated sufficiently to be able to decipher only disconnected fragments of written language, dyslexic. Failure to read through lack of educational opportunity is usually, however, called illiteracy to distinguish it from dyslexia. A dyslexic may be illiterate, but an illiterate need not necessarily be dyslexic—unless, indeed, the very process of aging beyond a critical developmental period before learning to read itself induces dyslexia. It would be interesting to know if, among illiterate octogenarians receiving reading instruction for the first time, dyslexia is more frequent than among juveniles.

* The author is supported in full-time research by Grant No. M-1557, the National Institute of Mental Health, United States Public Health Service.

When there is some record of the degree of reading achievement once attained, it is not difficult to recognize the existence of post-traumatic or degenerative dyslexia. In the case of developmental dyslexia, it is also not too difficult to recognize the syndrome in older and teen-age children whose failure to profit from reading instruction is severe and quite out of harmony with other developmental achievements.

In point of fact, developmental dyslexia is usually defined as a failure which is severe and which is specifically in reading. The failure either does not apply to the hearing and speaking of language, or else affects these activities only slightly. The same is true for other deficiencies, as in calculation, mechanics, music, and so forth.

Pragmatically, this definition of dyslexia is all well and good. In schools it provides an effective practical basis for screening pupils of like disability for special instruction. From the point of view of understanding etiological principles, the definition is not satisfactory. Whatever specific dyslexia may eventually be analyzed to be, there is no reason to presuppose that it always occurs in isolation. It may, in fact, be part and parcel of a larger entity of cognitional incompetence or mental deficiency. Moreover, it may also be so severe as to greatly impair general mental efficiency and so produce a condition analogous to that pseudofeeblemindedness, so-called, which is secondary to psychotic disturbance, and also analogous to cerebrocognitional language and communication defects of aphasic type, or even to peripheral hearing loss.

At the present time specific dyslexia is ordinarily considered quite separate from mental deficiency and generalized retardation of learning. In dyslexia research, if not in classroom practice, the distinction should not be hard and fast, for the mechanisms of disability in the two groups may prove to have considerable overlap.

Severe specific dyslexia and generalized mental deficiency both delay the acquisition of literacy. But they do more. They permanently limit the level of literacy finally attained. In the case of specific dyslexia, the degree of final impairment of literacy appears to be inversely related to the IQ and to the caliber of mental abilities not dyslexically affected. It is possible for a child with an

IQ above 130 to be, by the age of ten, severely impeded and re-tarded specifically in reading, relative to his other academic achieve-ments. Yet this same child may well be reading better than a non-dyslexic contemporary with an IQ of 80. With tuition in remedial reading, the child of high IQ may readily reach the level average for his age. Such normality is deceptive, however, for the youngster ought to attain a superior reading level in keeping with his IQ. It is not known, in cases of this type, whether the reading deficit of the early years eventually becomes overcome, with ultimate achievement of superiority in reading. In other words, it cannot be definitely stated that such a case is simply a special instance of a "slow bloomer" with ultimate full flowering.

Slow blooming presents a special problem for school administra-tions in the matter of reading readiness at the age when schooling is begun. To differentiate the slow bloomers from the dyslexically handicapped is a major problem awaiting research.

Slow blooming is a form of temporary delay or retardation of literacy which in many instances, probably the majority, is self-correcting. Without proper teaching, however, it may become a self-perpetuating retardation.

Self-perpetuating retardation that can be reversed is encountered in those cases of a generalized learning block associated with, and secondary to, chronic problems of psychological maladjustment and adversity. It is not yet clearly established, one way or the other, whether this type of secondary learning block can be specific for reading, leaving the other school studies unaffected.

The concept of a secondary learning-block, specific to reading, demands a consideration of the phenomenon of a specific reading block in a person already fluent in reading. Such a reading block may, in fact, be not only specific to the activity of reading, but also restricted to certain types of books, as in the case of a nun who "went blank" when trying to read the Bible, or a psychoanalyst in training who became unable to concentrate on his assignments in Freud. This kind of hysterical, dissociative reading problem clini-cally presents a quite different syndrome from dyslexia.

The dissociative "reading black-out" is the syndrome to which the psychoanalytic theory of defective reading might best apply, if it applies at all. In psychoanalytic theory, a reading block is attributed to the sexual significance of the looking that reading involves. The reading block is thus an extension of an avoidance of looking. It is considered related to hostility toward the parent of the same sex and to inadequate identification with this parent.

Walters, Van Loan and Crofts (1961) conducted a quite ingenious experiment to see if these psychoanalytic propositions might also apply to low reading achievement in school children. The results were inconclusive and such differences as were found could be quite well accounted for by other than psychoanalytic hypotheses.

Rationale for the Existence of the Syndrome of Specific Dyslexia

Though there was extended discussion at the conference pertaining to the characteristics of specific dyslexia, there was no questioning the existence of the syndrome.

Medicine and pedagogy have been slow to come together in joint study of problems of mutual interest. On the one hand, there is still a substantial pedagogical tradition that sees all reading retardation as a problem of defective instruction and there is keen argument over the phonic versus the sight-recognition methods of teaching reading. On the other hand, there is a growing body of medical opinion that some cases of reading failure represent not poor instruction; not a dearth of motivation from an impoverished, illiterate family and neighborhood background; not emotional blockage; not generalized intellectual deficit; and not ocular disability. Rather these cases represent a specific disability of cognitional or gnosic function in written language and communication that resembles the aphasic sequelae of some brain injuries.

In recent years, the greatest impetus to this point of view has come from the study of hearing and speech disorders. Refinements of diagnostic method, notably in the application of the conditional-reflex method to the detection of auditory perception and discrimination, have pointed the way. They have shown that there are many patients whose peripheral organs of hearing, namely the ears and auditory nerves, are perfectly intact. Yet, these patients are unable to unscramble the flow of sounds that reach the brain so that they have the same order, pattern and meaning as they had on former occasions and as they continue to have for other people. These patients have a developmental, central auditory receptive defect. It is quite analogous to the impairment of comprehension of speech that one finds after injury to certain areas of the brain from, say, a stroke or penetrating wound.

The types of interference with the communicational function following damage to the brain are quite extraordinary in their variety and above all in their specificity. In the usual classification, they are subdivided as being primarily receptive or expressive. Receptive disorders are specified as involving chiefly auditory (receptive aphasia), visual (agnosia), or tactile (astereognosia) input. Output disorders are specified as linguistic (expressive aphasia) and motor-gestural (apraxia). Other instances of specificity are alexia, agraphia, acalculia, nominal aphasia, semantic or syntactic aphasia, and so on.

Geschwind's paper gives striking evidence of how the reading function may be destroyed by a brain lesion. Paralleling receptive aphasias having to do with the spoken word, these posttraumatic reading cases logically suggest a parallel inference, namely, that dyslexia may exist also as a developmental syndrome for which no brain lesion has, as yet, been demonstrated.

Traumatic and Developmental Dyslexia Compared

Traumatic injuries to the infantile or juvenile brain do not produce the same functional effects and symptoms as do the same injuries to a brain that has already matured in function. There were several occasions during the conference discussion when attention was drawn to this fact. The immature brain has greater plasticity which allows it to compensate for injury, both through the use of substitutive pathways and through greater ease of localizing language functions in the nondominant hemisphere if their normal location in the dominant hemisphere is damaged.

The principle that injury to an immature organ has a different phenomenological effect than injury to a mature one has wide application in biology and medicine—in the effects of juvenile and adult hypothyroidism for example. Thus one does not expect dyslexia after trauma in people who once could read competently to be phenomenologically the same as dyslexia that shows up developmentally after known early brain injury. But it is usually the case that developmental dyslexia appears without demonstrable early brain injury. As it is, there is at present no systematic knowledge on relationships between the incidence of dyslexia and of various childhood ailments that are known to affect the brain. Kawi and Pasamanick (1959) found a statistical relationship between reading disorder and abnormal conditions during the pregnancy and childbirth, especially toxemia of pregnancy and bleeding during pregnancy. They found a similar relationship between these same pregnancy complications and stillbirths, neonatal deaths, cerebral palsy, epilepsy and behavior disorders.

Though the two conditions cannot be equated, there is much of pertinence to developmental dyslexia to be learned from the study of posttraumatic dyslexia, namely in the specificity of impairment possible in these latter cases. The language and communicational function may suffer generalized disablement, but it may also be selectively interfered with, for, to an astonishing degree, the components of communication can be autonomous in the organization and function of the brain.

Wepman presented one of his own cases which is aptly illustrative at this point. This is the case of a man who was left severely impaired following a stroke—blind, then partially blind, color-blind, agnosic, unable to recognize much that was within the field of vision; and unable to write though his ability to read was unimpaired. With time he made improvement and his skill with calculation returned to the point where he could resume his occupation as an auditor. He had difficulty in the recognition of only one type of visual image—that of the common life object. He could recognize geometric forms even when enlarged on a screen. He had no difficulty with language, or with auditory signals. He managed life quite well, except for needing an escort to compensate for his agnosia of objects. Then, without the escort one day, he failed to recognize a bus for what it was, walked in front of it, and was killed.

Geschwind's paper makes clear, as did the discussion that followed it, that the localization of language functions and subfunctions is no simple matter of areas. One must think rather in three dimensions as of an edifice composed of many different pavilions built adjacent to, on top of, and inside of one another, each of them webbed to the other in an interconnection of looped circuits up and down, side to side, front to back, and across the surface. In so ramified a system, it is possible for a lesion to be highly specific in its effect, blocking, say, the visual language recognition routes, but sparing enough compensatory, detour routes so as to not even interfere with writing, with object recognition and naming, and with spoken and heard language (Casey and Ettlinger, [1960]).

In developmental dyslexia, as in the posttraumatic variety, one encounters much individual variation as to the extent of involvement of aspects of the communication and related functions other than reading. Saunders' paper gives illustrative examples of this variability, as do the papers by Benton and Zangwill.

Diagnosis of the Syndrome of Developmental Dyslexia

The obvious criterion of reading retardation is that a child is not able to score at the reading achievement level proper to its age and years of instruction. It is a simple matter to identify reading retardation, but far from simple to make the differential diagnosis of specific dyslexia. This theme reappeared many times in the conference discussion. Schiffman drew attention to the problem in identifying pupils for special reading services in schools. Newbrough and Kelly encountered the problem in their epidemiological study, since the school records and appraisals they used identified only the degree of a pupil's reading retardation. The problem reappears in Prechtl's research. Children with his newly discovered choreiform syndrome may be handicapped in school learning and retarded in reading as in other subjects. There was no evidence, however, that their condition promoted specific reading handicaps.

The fact of the matter is that no one has yet devised a foolproof way of diagnosing specific dyslexia. There is seldom argument about extreme cases, like those presented by Saunders, with their extreme handicap and their telltale errors. The problem arises in less severe cases. Rabinovitch said that in his clinic they have often found themselves making double-barreled diagnoses like: "secondary retardation with a touch of primary disability."

The diagnostic problem is even more acute when, among prereaders and beginning readers, one would like to differentiate a prognosis of specific dyslexia from one of "late blooming" or of generalized learning block. To a significant degree the problem hinges around the fact that no one has as yet uncovered any telltale sign or group of signs that are exclusive to the syndrome of specific dyslexia and are not found in other conditions of reading retardation. In fact, the special errors and failures characteristic of specific dyslexia can all be found, albeit in much attenuated form, in the beginning reader, especially if he is tested to the limit of his ability and achievement, or under conditions of duress.

It is not at all rare in psychological medicine, nor in other branches of medicine, that a disease should have no unique identifying sign, that uniqueness being in the pattern of signs that appear in contiguity. Out of context, each sign might also be encountered in other diseases, or, in different intensities, in the healthy. Specific dyslexia is no exception in this respect. A good example of this is the matter of reversals and translocations of letters, discussed below.

Of course there is no foretelling what new testing methods may uncover. Adaptation of a conditional-reflex technique to testing visual discrimination, as auditory discrimination is tested in hearing and speech clinics, is one possibility. Even so, it still seems very likely that tests will for a long time to come be testing failure to achieve that which is normally expected at a given stage of development, as is the case in hearing and speech tests. Thus it appears that the diagnosis of specific dyslexia will continue not to depend on a single telltale sign, or signs, but on the clinical appraisal of the whole configuration of symptoms and test findings.

From the point of view of case management the diagnostic obstacles are not as great as they may seem. Whatever the etiology of reading retardation, the known principles and stages of therapy are the same. One does not force the young child to go beyond its proper level of reading readiness, and by the same token one does not hold the child back, either! Reading tuition is individualized, scholastically and psychotherapeutically, as much as economics permit. A variety of pedagogical techniques is tested to find the more successful. Subject to economic considerations, the special teaching program is extended as long as the student needs it and derives profit from it.

Directional Orientation

Reversal and translocation of letters are examples of persistent dyslexic traits not peculiar to dyslexics. Those errors are notoriously common among all beginners in reading and writing. Usually, however, they are eliminated after a brief history of only weeks or months. Yet the potentiality for reversals is never eliminated. The adult in typing—even the professional typist—continues to make reversals when working at high speed or under conditions of fatigue and duress. Proofreading is another example, especially when the reader is working on his own manuscript. He misses reversals and translocations in abundance, reading the word as it should be without adverting to the error that his mind has automatically corrected for him. The dyslexic individual is not unique in making reversals and translocations, but he is unique in making so many of them and for so long a time.

The errors of reversal and translocation need experimental investigation from the point of view of the psychology of camouflage.

W–A–S is a camouflage of S–A–W to the dyslexic, and he is fooled
just as easily as by a jungle suit camouflaged by jungle foliage.
A very basic point in the psychology of perception and concept
formation is involved here. In developmental cognition, the human
child makes two achievements simultaneously. On the one hand
he builds up an inventory of what, among the parade of patterns
of figures against backgrounds that reach his retina and his other
senses, must be classified as separate entities. On the other hand
he builds up paradigms of how many different sensory patterns an
object may make and still be the same object. Thus a cup is a cup
whether it is sitting or hanging, upright or inverted, seen from
below or above one's eyes, with the handle to the left, right, front
or rear, and even when it is lying smashed in pieces. Not so with
characters of the alphabet like b and d, p and q! And not so
with the arrangement of the alphabetic characters in words. Their
positional sequence and not their mere presence is then of utmost
importance: w–o–r–d–y is not the same as r–o–w–d–y, but they
may be to a dyslexic, since the same five letters are in each.

Success with the alphabet in reading and writing requires the
reader to override the principle of constancy that usually applies,
namely that the significance of a something remains constant
despite inconstancy of the configuration of the perceptual sign,
as in the cup paradigm, above. A cup turned around is still a cup,
but a b turned sideways is a d, and turned head to toe is a p
and turned both ways at the same time is a q (and nearly a 9
and a g). The dyslexic has the greatest difficulty in permanently
and routinely allocating all this specificity of significance to an alter-
ation not of shape but simply of directional orientation.

In the past a good deal has been written and said about mirror
reversals in dyslexia, along with speculations about the dominance
of the right or the left hemisphere of the brain. A much misunder-
stood point in this context is that mirror reversal is not only a left-
to-right reversal as it is when you stand in front of a mirror and try
to write your name on your own forehead; it is also a near-and-far
reversal, as when you try to write at your desk looking not at the
page but its reflection in a mirror propped up in front of you. The
dyslexic makes the first kind of error when he makes a d for a b,

and the second when he make a p for a b. His problem is not one of left-right dominance but one of confusion about the direction of the optical image of a symbol in relation to the muscular "feel" of making it.

Make a test on yourself. Close your eyes and "tattoo" a word on a piece of paper held to your forehead. Write y o u. Take the card down and see that almost certainly you have written ∪ o ɣ. Yet you could swear that it felt as though you had written y o u. Why? Normally your hand goes out to write on a surface facing your eyes. The same thing would have happened had you tried to write on a wall behind your head. It would also have happened had you tried to put your hand through an open window and write on the outside of the glass. Then you would have seen through the transparent glass an image that looked properly readable to you, but seen from outdoors it would be mirror writing.

We are so used to writing on a surface facing the eyes that when we write on a surface that faces away from the eyes we automatically do so as though that surface were transparent and the eyes were seeing the message. In actual fact the visual image on the written surface is obverted concordantly with the obversion of the kinesthetic imagery from the writer's fingers, hand, and arm below the rotated elbow.

Obviously this double obversion of imagery, visual and kinesthetic, is related to the fact that there is an area of one's body from just below the chin, all over the head and neck and down the back to nearly the back of the knee which can never be seen by direct gaze. Every part of this area, except the back of the head and neck, can be touched only by rotating the arm at the elbow, as in shaving the face as contrasted with painting on a canvas. Now, all movements of the hands in relation to simultaneously perceived visual images are normally made in the same position as painting on canvas. Obversion of the forearm by rotation at the elbow is imperative specifically for actions performed on those parts of one's own body which one cannot see.

Although we can never see these actions we perform on ourselves, most of us apparently "visualize" them in imagination as if they were taking place out in front of our own eyes. Evidently the dyslexic has confusion and difficulty in the matter of body image for the parts of the body he can both see and feel and those he can only feel. Apparently he gets a feeling that he wrote y o u , as though on his own knee, when in fact he wrote ∪ o ɣ , as though on his own forehead; or that he read w ᴆ ƨ when the book in fact read s ɑ w .

It is this confusion between visual and body images that seems to underlie the difficulties of directional orientation that have been noted as a characteristic of dyslexics. Their problem is not a simple one of right-left confusion, though that may exist too. Nor is it only a matter of difficulty with perception of form in two dimensions. It is truly a three-dimensional *space-movement* perception problem, involving the relationship of the visual image to the body image in ahead and behind, toward and away-from, left and right and facing upward or downward.

Howes mentioned an experimental irony pertinent at this point. Sutherland (1960), studying visual discrimination in the octopus, found that the animals had special difficulty in discriminating right and left diagonals. The irony was that the experimenters had the same trouble and had to mark the backs of the cards, ® and Ⓛ . No wonder! The shape that appears thus, / , when held up to the experimenter's eyes becomes obverted to him, \ , when he turns the card round and holds it up to the octopus' gaze.

Another pertinent observation, made at the end of Howes's paper, is Kohler's finding regarding people wearing right-left reversal prisms. When the brain, accommodated to the wearing of prisms, makes the adjustment of correcting the reversal of images, it returns them all to their proper directional orientation, except the images of words, letters, and numbers. Possibly the tardiness of written symbols to be corrected is related to the fact that they are not only visual images in one's literate experience, but also kinesthetic ones, and therefore different from all the multitude of those visual images that are never actually created by one's own hand. Perhaps the paradox pointed out by Howes and Geschwind in Dejerine's famous case, namely that the patient did not become agnosic for visual objects but only for words, is related to this same fact. Maybe the patient's brain lesion destroyed some kinesthetic-visual-language pathways, leaving intact the kinesthetic-language pathways (the patient could write), as Geschwind has suggested, and the visual-language ones.

The relationship of directional orientation to body image raises the question of body image in relation to the finger agnosia described by Gerstmann in his syndrome of right-left disorientation, dysgraphia, dyscalculia, and finger agnosia. There is a tricky way of destroying the normal relation of visual to kinesthetic image of the fingers and so disturbing finger gnosia. Hold your palms facing you, with the forearms crossed. In an awkward movement that requires rotation of wrists, elbows and shoulders, bring the two palms together, thumb facing thumb and little finger facing little finger, the wrists still crossed. Lace the fingers of each hand into the corresponding interdigital spaces of the other. You now are quite likely, with eyes open or closed, to have difficulty in recognizing which finger was touched, or which one to move when given an instruction.

Dyslexia in Other Languages

There is a brief report from Kobe Medical College on dyslexia in a twelve-year-old Japanese boy by the Japanese neuropsychiatrists, Kuromaru and Okada (1961). The Japanese use two methods of writing, the ancient Chinese ideographic method (Kanji script) and a more recent, syllabary, phonetic system resembling our own alphabetic system (Kana script). Kuromaru and Okada reported that their patient had great difficulty with the syllabary, Kana script. He was unable to break it up into its sounds and letters correctly, and unable to assemble the syllabary elements into their proper units, words. By contrast, though the Kanji ideographs were difficult to learn, the patient's recognition of the meaning of the ideograph was usually easier than that of a Kana word.

Recall briefly the example of the cup and its handle in the foregoing section. A Kanji ideograph is rather like a cup. Upside down

or in mirror reversal, it probably has a much greater chance than
the parallel Kana word of being recognized for what it is.

It is true that the student has to learn to differentiate one ideograph from another, some of them closely similar. But this is a
different task from recognizing differences among an equal number
of Kana words, some of them also closely similar, and all of them
constructed of the same 50 alphabetic characters.

One has heard claims that developmental dyslexia does not exist
in Spanish-speaking schools because the language is so perfectly
phonetic. Bauza, Carbonell, Drets and Escuder (1962) have shown,
however, that developmental dyslexia does exist in Uruguay.
Phonetic regularity is of no help to the child who cannot remember
the name and sound of each letter, and it does not totally abolish
the problems of mirror writing and reading. Dr. Ernesto Pollitt
has told me of a case of traumatic aphasia with dyslexia in a six-
teen-year-old boy from Lima. The patient was able to decipher
and pronounce short words without comprehending their meaning,
but he was unable to decipher long words of six syllables or more.

For experimental purposes, it would be of interest to try teaching a totally phonetic script to a group of dyslexic children, and
an ideographic or rebus script to another group.

Inventory Memory and Concept Memory

Consider the experiment of learning a picture vocabulary in
which there is perfect correlation between the pictorial image and
its signification. The image is never used with any other meaning,
and the meaning is never represented by any other image— O
always means ring and nothing else, and ring is always represented
by O and by nothing else. Further, each image remains unchanged in its significance, like the cup mentioned earlier, regardless of positional changes—backward, upsidedown, slanted—or
other changes as of color, shading, or fragmentation. In the technical language of information theory, there is no noise in the
system.

The learner of this picture vocabulary has a twofold memory task: to build up an inventory of the different symbols, and to develop a concept of the identity and constancy of each symbol despite variations in position, color, and suchlike.

Compare by contrast the problem of learning our alphabetic and number script. The necessity of building an inventory of symbols remains, but the constancy concept of each symbol is hedged in with all manner of provisos. The symbols do not change meaning with changes of color or density; but some of them do change meaning by reason of changed directional orientation:

| b d | p q | f t | 6 9 | *n u* |

or of having fragments omitted:

h n	o c	a o	e c	˅ m n
n r	w v	I r	*b l*	*w u*
Q O	L I	B 3	8 S	Z 7

or a combination of both:

| A V | t r | *j i* | *b a* | *p a* |

To confound matters even further, the upper and lower case of both cursive and printing scripts give each letter variant forms, some of them not even remotely resembling one another. In addition, the various type fonts add not only extra minor variations, but some further radical departures as well.

The visual inconstancy permitted and not permitted each letter-concept in the alphabet is, therefore, extremely capricious and illogical—and all of this independently of the phonetic irregularities involved in translating the letter into sounds!

It is not therefore too surprising that dyslexics turn out to be people who also have difficulty in establishing concepts. Saunders makes reference to this fact; Rabinovitch and his Michigan associates have developed the Hawthorn Concepts Scale for use with dyslexics. A specific conceptual problem for some dyslexics is in color recognition and naming.

The dyslexic's conceptual confusion does not end with the alphabet but is further compounded by the vagary with which the shapes of letters are assembled into words. The word is a visual image that takes on meaning not by reason simply of the presence its component images, but by reason of their sequential arrangement in space. Reversal or rearrangement of the same few letters totally destroys the conceptual constancy and identity of the entity, that is, the word. True, conceptual constancy is not destroyed if a whole word is turned upside down or held up to a mirror—with practice one can soon learn to read such pages. But the constancy of sequential arrangement of letters one after another is the *sine qua non* of a word's identity. So basic is this rule that exceptions to it have an element of surprise, as in a palindrome—MADAM I'M ADAM—which reads the same backward and forward. Again, letter order is the basis of parlor games, as in the anagrammatic transpositions—*shoe* to *hose; except* to *expect; shiek* to *hikes*—and other scrambled word puzzles.

Acquiring a reading vocabulary therefore is basically a feat of building up an inventory of visual patterns all made up out of the same 26 alphabetic components and distinguished from one another only by reason of the sequential arrangement of the components. The learner, must form a concept of each word as a symbol which retains a constant identity despite variations in position, size, color, or script-shape, but which completely loses identity if fragmented and reassembled in different sequential order.

Acquiring an English-reading vocabulary is a feat of visual inventory memory, but not so much so as it would be in acquiring an inventory of nonalphabetic, picture-vocabulary. Our spelling is phonetic, despite exasperating inconsistencies, so that the learner is permitted to translate the visual images into an auditory, phonic system which has its own rules and irregularities of symbol identity and constancy. The advantage of this is that sufficient regularities exist in the phonetic system to permit recognition of the component syllables in totally unfamiliar words, and so allow the entire word to be figured out phonetically. Thus the size of the phonic inventory the learner must acquire is smaller than the visual inventory for the same number of words drawn exclusively in picture vocabulary.

Pedagogically it is economical to use both phonic and visual-recognition methods of teaching reading. When only the visual method is used, many children with competence in concept formation evolve their own concepts of phonetic identities and constancies. When only the phonic method is used, it cannot apply to phonetically irregular words. Moreover, all reading vocabulary eventually becomes sight-recognition vocabulary for the accomplished, speedy reader. He acquires a vast inventory of words each one of which is recognizable on sight, almost instantaneously.

The prominence of inventory memory in acquiring reading vocabulary is rather well illustrated in two of my own recent cases. One is a case of a girl with the IQ of a mental defective and relative hyperlexia. The other is a case of a precocious boy with a superior IQ who has taught himself to read.

Case No. 1. This is a case of a girl of thirteen with a history of congenital hypothyroidism (which typically impairs the IQ) diagnosed at the age of two months but undertreated with a suboptimal thyroid dosage until the girl was seven. At seven and a half, her Wechsler Intelligence Scale for Children IQs were: Verbal 69, Performance 62, Full 62; and at eight they were 65, 60, and 59 respectively. Nonetheless she demonstrated, when she was eight and a half, a dramatically surprising ability to read from the first-grade reader, after one year at school; she was not parroting, but read with good word recognition and comprehension. At the age of 12 years and 11 months, her WISC IQs were 76, 61, 66; the highest scaled score was 8, on Digit Span, the other Verbal Scaled Scores ranging between 5 and 7, the Performance between 3 and 6. Her rating on the Benton Visual Retention Test was average for her age. A year later the parents gave anecdotal evidence of the girl's memory. She could recall all telephone numbers and addresses used by the family, all the hymns and their page numbers in the church hymnal, and all the arithmetic tables. At school she had passed out of special classes into a regular seventh grade and was obtaining grades between 70 and 80. Her reading and general scholastic level was thus far above her IQ and corresponded with her inventory memory.

Case No. 2. This boy was not recognized as particularly unusual when he entered first grade at the age of 6 years 3 months except that he passed reading tests for the fourth grade. At the age of 6 years and 4 months his WISC IQs were: Verbal 110, Performance 115, Full 114; and a month later, they were 121, 122, and 124 respectively (different place and tester). On the repeat test, the verbal scaled scores ranged from 12 to 14, except for 16 on Similarities and 17 on Digit Span. The performance scaled scores ranged from 14 to 15, except for Coding, which was 9 (on which subtest he lost points on the time limit because restless and slow). While being tested, the boy often stopped to repeat entire TV commercials for toys, verbatim.

The boy's own preference, to demonstrate his reading, was to find in magazines advertisements of products familiar to him on television. These he could read fluently and with perfect word recognition, though subsequent attempts to write them were riddled with guessed, quasi-phonetic spelling. Sight reading of *Life* magazine captions was not fluent, but quite adequate in comprehension and with some excellent phonic decipherments of long words.

The mother first noticed the boy's ability to read when he was about three. In the supermarket he would recognize labels and slogans he had seen on TV commercials, and would read these same words in magazine ads. This learning was spontaneous. There were no older siblings or relatives to copy. The parents did not particularly encourage reading in the home, but provided plenty of the usual children's books. They were not well educated themselves, were young and of low income. The mother appeared to be of superior IQ.

The boy had a detailed memory for much that he could read in his books at home. Recently he had surprised his mother with enumerations of encyclopedic facts about birds, from his children's encyclopedia.

High IQ alone is inadequate to explain this boy's precocious reading. An exceptional inventory memory seems to have played an important role especially in his exceptional sight-recognition vocabulary.

Visile and Audile Types

In the final analysis, a reading vocabulary is an inventory of immediately recognizable visual images. Phonic analysis can enable one to say a written word, even a totally unfamiliar word in a totally unfamiliar language, such as from the perfectly phonetic scripts of the Polynesian dialects. In English, phonic analysis is a steppingstone to visual recognition by way of auditory recognition. Eventually the visual image becomes autonomous and the act of reading is an act of recognizing visual images.

During the conference, there was some mention of Charcot's hypothesis that there are visile and audile types. It is quite conceivable that the dyslexic is a person who has difficulty not only in establishing the necessary lexical concepts, visual and auditory, as discussed above, and in relating the visual and phonic image, but who also is in some manner a nonvisile cognitional type. He is perhaps a person weak in visual imagery and visual memory of all types, the opposite of the person with eidetic imagery and photographic memory. There is far too little known of imagistic and cognitional types in psychology, and pitifully little attention given to the problem. There is plenty of room for investigation here, generally, and specifically in relation to dyslexia. What about the dreaming of dyslexics, for example? Waggenheim (1960) reported a study on first memories of accidents in dyslexic children, but this was a study of content, not type of memory imagery.

Logically, one may expect that a specific visile deficit may exist in isolation. In this case the person would show few or no signs of aphasic disturbance in speaking and listening, only agnosic disturbances of reading and writing (like reading "sketchy" for "sticky"—see other examples in Saunder's paper). A visile deficit coexistent with an audile one would show up as a severe disturbance of all language. Conceivably one might also find praxile (tactile or kinesthetic) deficits which would interfere with the input and output for touch language and writing, e.g.; as used by the blind. It is well established that the handwriting of dyslexics is in many instances severely defective—one is tempted to say dyspraxic.

In contrast with the concept of imagistic and cognitional types, Birch in his paper raises the very important concept of developmental and maturational changes in the discrimination and competition of imagery and perception, through the eyes, ears, and sense of touch.

Cerebral Dominance

In the loose thinking of times past, cerebral dominance has been implicated in dyslexia in relation to mirror writing and right-left reversals. Zangwill's paper gives a definitive statement of contemporary knowledge. The reader is also referred to the proceedings of a cerebral dominance conference at Johns Hopkins in April, 1961 (Mountcastle [1962]).

There are two purposes in reopening the topic at this point, of which the first is to refer to two cases of stroke mentioned by Geschwind in the discussion of Zangwill's paper—those of Pitres (1884) and of Nielsen (1946). They both illustrate the fact that people with right, instead of the normal, left, cerebral dominance may be trained to write with not the left but the right hand, and in spite of this, the right cerebral dominance will be retained (Ettlinger, Jackson, and Zangwill [1956]). For a right-handed person, the cerebral dominance is usually in the left hemisphere. The persistence of cerebral speech dominance despite contrary manual training is not too surprising when one thinks of instrumentalists whose left hands get intensive training without, presumably, making them right-brained.

The second purpose of reopening the topic of cerebral dominance is to point out that the information the foregoing cases and Zangwill's paper furnish is completely incompatible with current faddist therapies of dyslexia on the basis of hypotheses of cerebral dominance (Delacato [1959]). Scientifically speaking, it is far too premature to be applying hypotheses of cerebral dominance to methods of treatment. What these hypotheses need, above all else, is to be tested experimentally, and in controlled observation, for validity.

Vision

Ocular and optical defects are of negligible dyslexic significance. Even when severe and uncorrected, such defects are usually sufficiently overcome to permit the learning of reading. When too severe to permit reading, then these defects, if uncorrected, induce not specific dyslexia, but generalized academic underachievement.

Apropos of vision, it is timely to mention that specific dyslexia is one of the group of learning failures that sometimes comes within the purvue of a faddist therapy that is currently enjoying considerable vogue, generally under optometric auspices (Getman [1958]). This therapy is derived from a doctrine of the interrelatedness of motor, auditory, linguistic and visual maturation—with particular emphasis on visuomotor or visuopostural relatedness. The fallacy of this faddism is that it takes hypotheses which, quite conceivably, are valid principles of development (Harmon [1958]) and applies them, prematurely and untested, as principles of training and treatment, with unjustified reliance on disproved assumptions concerning that old psychological war horse, the transfer of training.

What is needed in the place of prematurely applied visual theories is more basic investigation of vision and seeing as developmental processes prerequisite to reading. There is, for example, the recent work by Goins (1958) and Frostig (1961) on visual discriminatory skills and reading readiness. One important finding of Goins was the negation of Renshaw's claim (1945) that tachistoscopic training in *Gestalt* perception can improve general visual perceptual ability. There are two laboratories, that of Held ([1961]; Held & Bossom [1961]) at Brandeis University, and of Riesen (1958; 1961) at the University of Chicago, where experiments on sensory deprivation, visual form perception and motor performance in animals are of basic importance in the psychology of vision. This comparative experimental approach may turn out to be of great significance to the psychology of reading and is well worth watching.

There is an important relationship between vision and cerebral dominance by way of the visual cortex. In the neurological literature there appear several papers dealing with the effects of injury to the right and the left visual cortex (Hécaen, de Ajuriaguerra, and Massonnet [1951]; Hécaen, de Ajuriaguerra, and David [1952]; Ettlinger, Warrington, and Zangwill [1957]; McFie and Zangwill [1960]; Piercy, Hécaen, and de Ajuriaguerra [1960]). Injury to the visual cortex on one side produces loss of vision over part of the retinal field of each eye, namely on the same side of both retinas, the loss for each eye being on the same side as the brain injury. This loss is not a simple matter of blindness on the retina, but appears to represent unilateral agnosia or neglect of visual stimuli, that is, unilateral incapacity to pay attention. Thus a patient with a right-sided brain lesion will have the *right* retinas and *left* visual fields affected. He may draw a house with the left side missing and be unable to recognize that something is missing. In relation to the directional problem in dyslexia, it is of great interest to know that visual attention has this characteristic of being lateralized. Cohn (1961b) showed a relationship between this lateralized impairment of attention to space and dyscalculia, notably in long multiplication.

Hormones

Dyslexia may occur in children who also have some or other endocrine disease. Specific dyslexia is not, however, a symptomatic characteristic of any of these diseases, which statement I make on the authority of ten years of clinical experience in the psychology of pediatric endocrine disorders. In particular, dyslexia is not a characteristic of hypothyroidism. Even a low IQ is not universal in congenital hypothyroidism, which is notorious for its impairment of intelligence.

It would seem unnecessary to mention these facts, except that yet another faddism has appeared in the treatment of dyslexia (Smith and Carrigan [1959]) involving thyroid and other medications, on the basis of improbable and improperly tested hypotheses.

Sex Differences

Newbrough and Kelly found a ratio of three boys to two girls among the retarded readers they studied. Prechtl had a ratio of two boys to one girl in his sample of children with the choreiform syndrome. In specific dyslexia, the ratios may vary from sample to sample, but it is a unanimous finding that the male incidence is twice that of the female, if not more. This same lopsidedness turns up in the incidence figures for generalized underachievement, and does not apply only to reading failure. The lopsidedness appears again in delinquency figures. Moreover, as mentioned in Wepman's paper, there is a good deal of overlap between delinquency and academic underachievement, reading failure included, with no clear evidence as to which is cart and which is horse (Margolin, Roman, and Harari [1955]).

It is quite impossible at the present time to account for the differential sex ratio in the incidence of dyslexia. One is tempted to speculate on the fact that the sex ratio of live births is 106 boys to 100 girls; and even on the fact that the embryo deprived of sex glands before the reproductive system has differentiated always develops morphologically as a female, regardless of chromosomal status (Jost, 1954). Life expectancy is shorter for males than females. The sexual behavior disorders have a higher incidence in males than females. And so on. Evidently it is more hazardous to be a male, as the actuarial tables for automobile insurance show —at least to be an adolescent male.

The predominance of males with dyslexia is not related to any known disorders of sex hormone functioning; nor can it be attributed, on the basis of current endocrine knowledge and research techniques, to differences in hormone levels.

As with hormones, so also with chromosomes. The new technique of visualizing and counting chromosomes within the cells (Ferguson-Smith, [1961]; Sohval [1961]) has revealed no suggestion so far of a connection between chromosomal aberration and dyslexia. Some chromosomal disorders, however, do have a definite affinity with mental deficiency.

There is one sex difference that pertains to vision, namely that males more than females seem to be erotically responsive to visual stimuli (Money [1961]). In the strange economy of nature, it is not impossible, albeit wildly conjectural, that there is somewhere a connection between this sex difference in response to visual erotic stimuli and the sex difference in response to the visual stimuli of language.

Another quite wildly conjectural sex-difference hypothesis can be derived from some speculations of David B. Lynn (1961). Lynn suggests that infant girls acquire their sex-role identity by direct imitation of the mother; whereas infant boys, who spend more hours with the mother than the father, acquire their sex-role identity at second hand and, instead of directly imitating anyone, they have to restructure the field and abstract general principles. It has already been pointed out that acquiring a reading vocabulary is very much an inventory-building task rather than one of abstracting general principles. Conceivably then, girls, as a group, are by reason of their sexual identification better practiced in inventory building than are boys.

Reading Epilepsy

In some cases of dyslexia there may be positive EEG findings (Kennard, Rabinovitch, and Wexler [1952]), but in developmental dyslexia a positive EEG is not a routine expectation. It is a point of quite considerable, though isolated, interest, therefore, that in certain extremely rare cases the act of reading can induce an epileptic seizure. The syndrome was first described by Bickford, Whelan, Klass and Corbin in 1956. Two cases of primary reading epilepsy, with a review and bibliography, are given by Baxter and Bailey (1961). The seizure may appear in association with silent reading, but more likely with oral reading. The first signs are involuntary opening of the jaw and jaw clicking or snapping. There may be repetition of the syllable being pronounced. The full seizure may be aborted by cessation of reading. The patients do not have seizures under other circumstances and their neurological examinations are normal. The EEG is normal during the resting state but may show diffuse paroxysmal activity when jaw-opening movements are provoked by reading. Baxter and Bailey suggested that impulses from the muscles of the face and eyes during reading, especially under concentration, are important in precipitating the seizure.

Research Directions

The concluding discussion of the conference was on a dyslexia research program that might be carried out in a school system. Zangwill summed up the mood of the discussion by declaring in favor of investigative experimental studies and detailed clinical studies rather than large testing surveys. He pointed out that the syndromes of disease in medicine were not identified by large scale surveying, correlating, and factor-analyzing of symptoms and other data. There is a need for new tests that are more accurate and valid in the differential diagnosis of dyslexia. Experiment and clinical study is a prerequisite for the development of these tests.

2

Dyslexia: Its Phenomenology

ROGER E. SAUNDERS

Reading, the reconstruction of meaning behind printed symbols, is a necessary part of scholastic achievement if one is to communicate in a way other than by word of mouth. The need for adequacy in this area of communication has become increasingly demanding as compulsory education in many countries has increased.

Popular magazines and newspapers regularly contain some suggestions relative to the improvement of reading skills. The clamor for faster reading has even stimulated courses on television for the public. Reports of unbelievable speed in reading have spurred criticism of teaching techniques. Since success in reading is important, it becomes quite essential and appropriate that even greater attention should be given to those individuals who find it impossible to achieve the bare minimum of success in this task that the culture demands.

For over a century there have been startling accounts reported in medical journals of individuals who, after some type of cerebral trauma, lost their ability to read, with or without accompanying language deficits and disturbances. More recently it has been further discovered that, even in the absence of evidence of cerebral accident, some intellectually competent individuals exhibit a similar symptom of inability to learn to read. In this country Samuel T.

Orton (1937) stands out for his work in describing and defining the dyslexia syndrome. For other definitive statements, the reader is referred to Ranschburg (1928), Eustis (1947), Gillingham (1956), Hambright (1956), Hermann (1956), Thompson (1956), de Hirsch (1957), Rabinovitch (1959), Gallagher (1960), Silver and Hagin (1960), Cohn (1961a), O'Sullivan and Pryles (1962). Orton felt certain of the interrelatedness of all language functions and that children, in particular, with dyslexia were experiencing a developmental lag in acquiring language skills (Bender [1957], Wepman [1961]). Orton's unique contribution to education was that he inspired the development of pedagogical techniques for the remediation of dyslexia (Fernald [1943], Gillingham and Stillman [1956], Filbin [1957], Parker School [1957]).

The present president of the Orton Society, Mrs. Sally B. Childs, in a personal communication, estimated that, irrespective of etiology, twenty to thirty per cent of today's school population is retarded in reading. When identifying children suffering from reading retardation, one must keep in mind the possibility of numerous causative factors contributing to the problem. Heredity has been implicated (Hallgren [1950]). Children with clearly definable intellectual deficits, specific or general, constitute a large majority of any school's population of slow readers. On the other hand, it is altogether feasible that many children develop (or bring with them) personality problems which serve to hinder academic instruction from making its mark. Many other causes have been suggested, including environmental deprivation creating poor "readiness," absence of motivation, inadequate instruction, crowded classrooms, and somatic problems. However, in the absence of significant problems of the above type, there still remains a large percentage of children who cannot read on a level commensurate with their intelligence. For reasons unexplained, this percentage includes significantly more boys than girls. It is precisely these children whom we study for additional clues to their reading problems, for it is quite possible that they have dyslexia or a problem of such a specific nature as to merit the term, "specific language disability." One must seek beyond the numerical results of tests for the more subtle evidences of the specificity of this crippling disability.

There may be confusion over the exact definition of a retarded reader. To some, the criterion of "grade level," i.e., of reading achievement matching academic level, seems the best. Others feel that chronological age is the prime divider and that all data should be processed according to this base. There is no simple, single standard. It is important, when diagnosing dyslexia, to keep in mind the variability of the language function itself. Language in schools is more than just reading. It is also speaking, spelling, handwriting, oral and written expression—all of the communicative processes, including comprehension and interpretation. In the following paragraphs, some of these facets will be discussed as they apply to the dyslexic—child, adolescent or adult. The phenomena appear irrespective of age.

Usually the oral reading, for those who do have some word recognition skills, is done in a choppy, word-by-word manner much like that of the child that is just beginning to read, and utilizing an enormous amount of time for very simple tasks. It is not uncommon to find, particularly in dyslexic children below the fourth-grade level, regardless of their age, words read in reverse, for example, *was* as *saw*, *on* as *no*. A single letter may be reversed, as in *dig* for *big*. Often also there may be a transposition of some of the letters within a word, for example, *abroad* for *aboard*, *left* for *felt*, *how* for *who*. General confusion of words which have only a slightly different configuration abounds, for example, *through, though, thought*, and *quit, quiet, quite*. Repetition of words and phrases is common; and one gets the feeling that these children, though they have read the words accurately, do not comprehend the meaning of what they have just read aloud. Guesses are frequent, in view of the inability to handle the sounds-symbol system. They grasp for the meaning of unknown words on the basis of a few clues the rest of the printed material has furnished. It is also possible that, while working out a difficult word, there may be such a long pause that the meaning of the previously read words will escape them.

While oral reading is important, it is also quite revealing to listen to the spontaneous speech of children who experience some degree of dyslexia. For some, deviant speech (stuttering, lisping, stammering, cluttering) is quite noticeable; however, subtleties are important, for one might find in the dyslexic only slight and irregular problems of articulation (*wif* for *with*, *muvher* for *mother*), an unusually soft voice, or choppiness and nonfluency of speech. More confusing are the reversals of concepts, for example, *hostile* for *hospitable*, *floor* for *ceiling*, *go* for *stop*. Confusion of direction often is heard from these children, *east* for *west*, *up* for *down*, *under* for *over;* and time sequences also can be reversed: *first* for *last*, *now* for *later*, *seldom* for *often*. One child said, "The day after yesterday . . . I mean the day before tomorrow," when what he really meant was the day after tomorrow. Spoonerisms may be frequent (and the child will not know why others think him funny), as well as the scrambling of cultural clichés.

More is involved in language than reading and speaking. It is essential that the spelling and handwriting of children with this problem be critically scrutinized, for often errors fit into a fairly typical pattern. The penmanship may be characterized by poorly formed, irregular characters, and may lack a smooth, free-flowing evenness of style. The direction of the symbols may be reversed, and at times may be completely confused and illegible. In particular, letters which are similarly shaped but oppositely oriented are "crucial": p - g, b - d, q - g, u - n, and the printed *t* and *f*. Reversals of entire words (*was* and *saw*, *much* and *chum*, *the* and *eht*) or of letters within words (*trian* for *train*, *gril* for *girl*) are numerous in the dyslexic's script. The handwriting that is copied from a model may not be as inaccurate as spontaneous writing; however, clinical observations indicate that these children find copying from the blackboard, or from a printed exemplar, or note-taking to be difficult; and when they are under pressure, dyslexic symptoms occur with more frequency. Without specific help, written expression can be a laborious chore; and very often creative thoughts, when written down, are marred by inefficient spelling. The sensitive child who is victim of spelling errors may constrict his vocabulary when writing, and make his written work appear to be the product of immature thought processes by substituting, for example, "We went for something to eat" for "We went for groceries."

The naïve teacher may feel that a child learns only that which he is able to put on paper. This is not the case with children with this inability to express themselves in written work; and when measurement of achievement rests solely on this basis, then the child with dyslexia is unfairly judged.

Specimens of classroom work from dyslexic children are shown in Figures 1 to 5. These specimens demonstrate the dyslexic's problems of reversals, right-left confusion, transposition, omission, and deformed letters and syllables. Some of the words are undecipherable. By contrast with his misshapen words, a dyslexic's figure drawing may be quite well formed, as the one boy's drawing shows. All of the specimens were obtained from boys whose IQs were normal. Note that in several cases arithmetical ability was at, or near, the normal level for the child's grade in school, despite severe reading impairment.

As in neurological cases, so also in educational cases, there are extensive individual variations among dyslexics as to what they can and cannot do well scholastically. Thus, not all children who make errors in visual discrimination of letters exhibit speech-articulation difficulties. Again, some children can write perfectly formed letters, but their reading and spelling have the earmarks of dyslexia. Dyslexics may be adept at learning arithmetic, as indicated by scores on arithmetical-computational tests. There may or may not be failures in other symbol-association tasks, such as in learning musical notation, code, and scientific formulas.

Also variable among dyslexics are the various nonreading signs and symptoms that may go with the syndrome (Bender, [1956], Cohn, [1961a], Penfield and Roberts [1959]), many of which will be discussed in this book, namely, cerebral dominance, directionality, specific problems of vision and hearing, and problems of generalized physical clumsiness.

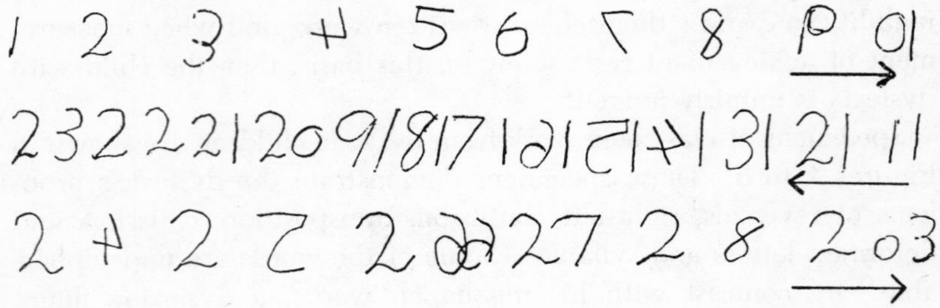

Figure 1. Reversals and left-right confusion in a boy half way through first grade. Age 6½. IQ 106.

Test List	Grade: 8th Age: 15-2 IQ: 93 Reading: 1.8 Spelling: 1.8 Arithmetic: 4.8	Grade: 3rd Age: 8-7 IQ: 119 Reading: 2.9 Spelling: 2.8 Arithmetic: 3.3	Grade: Sp. Ed. Age: 8-8 IQ: 93 Reading: 0 Spelling: 1.3 Arithmetic: 2.2	Grade: 4th Age: 9-5 IQ: 115 Reading: 3.6 Spelling: 3.3 Arithmetic: 4.4
cat	Cat	cat	ta C	cat
in	in	in	in	in
go	go	go	o g	go
man	nam	man	nar	man
will	will	wlle	I	will
and	and	and	dnd	and
boy	dog	d boy	boy	droy
make	nak	mak	Ca Ke	make
cut	k	cut		cut

Figure 2. Spelling lists of four dyslexic boys identified as to grade, age, IQ, and grade level of achievement in reading, spelling, and arithmetic.

Boy, 8th grade
Age, 13-7; IQ 108

Grade levels:
Reading   5.0
Spelling   4.5
Arithmetic 7.6

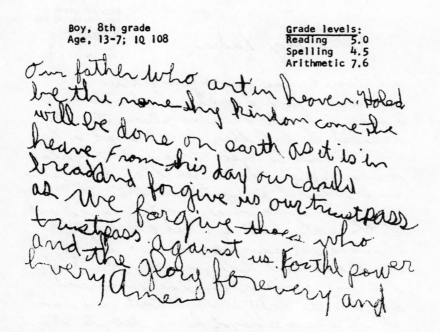

Figure 3. Classroom work of a dyslexic boy, assigned to write the Lord's Prayer from memory.

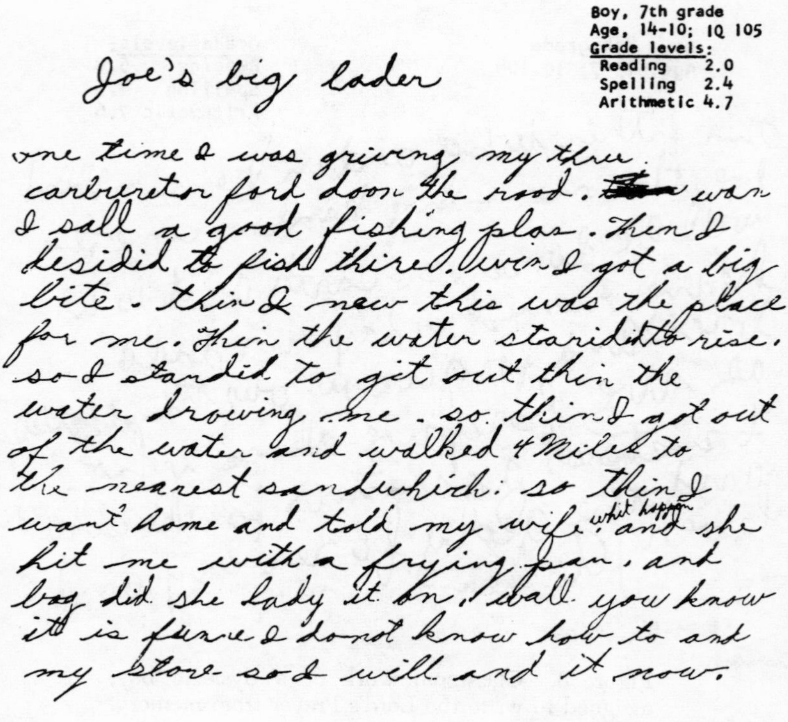

Boy, 7th grade
Age, 14-10; IQ 105
Grade levels:
  Reading   2.0
  Spelling   2.4
  Arithmetic 4.7

Joe's big lader

one time I was grieving my three.
carbureter ford down the road. the wan
I sall a good fishing plas . then I
desidid to fish thire. wen I got a big
bite . thin I new this was the place
for me. Then the water stariditto rise.
so I standid to git out thin the
water drowing me . so. thin I got out
of the water and walked 4 miles to
the nearest sandewhich: so thin I
want home and told my wife. *whit happen*and she
hit me with a frying pan. and
boy did she lady it on. wall you know
it is funie I donot know how to and
my store- so I will and it now.

Figure 4. English composition of a dyslexic boy. Assignment: Write a funny story.

Joe's Big [Lader]

One time I was driving my three
carburetor Ford down the road when
I saw a good fishing place. Then I
decided to fish there. When I got a big
bite, then I knew this was the place
for me. Then the water started to rise;
so I started to get out then, the
water drowning me. So then I got out
of the water and walked four miles to
the nearest sandwich. So then I
went home and told my wife what happened, and she
hit me with a frying pan, and
boy did she lay it on. Well, you know,
it is funny I do not know how to end
my story; so I will end it now.

Figure 5.   A line-by-line translation
of the story in Figure 4.

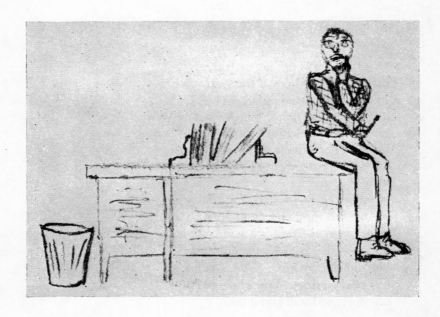

Figure 6.   Draw-a-Person Test. Done by the same boy who wrote "Joe's Big Lader." It is "a man sitting at a desk fixing to dictate a letter to his secretary. He's thinking about what he's going to say."

3

Dyslexia as an Educational Phenomenon: Its Recognition and Treatment

GILBERT SCHIFFMAN

The basic responsibility of the public school is to attempt to educate each pupil to the full extent of his capacity. In order to carry out this responsibility, it is necessary to provide special services and programs for pupils with problems which cannot be handled within the regular classroom context. For a multitude of reasons, there are pupils within any system who are not reading at a level in keeping with their capacity. (Authorities indicate that this figure ranges from twenty to forty per cent of the school's registration.) Ideally these pupils would be identified and remedied in the regular classroom by proper grouping and instruction. However, from experience we know this is not always possible or practical. For many of these children it is necessary that special reading programs be available at the elementary and secondary level to supplement the developmental program. Emphasis should be placed upon early identification and placement in the proper program before an individual's problem has become too complex.

A number of years ago educators realized that a total school reading program should provide three kinds of reading services:

developmental, corrective, and remedial. Perhaps we should digress for a moment and briefly define the three types. First, the developmental reading program involves systematic instruction at all school levels and in all content areas for those who are developing language abilities commensurate with their general capacity levels. This developmental phase is the responsibility of every teacher, affects all the pupils, is provided for in the regular curriculum and is a continuous process. Secondly, the corrective reading program must deal with those pupils who are able to comprehend the assigned material only after undue and laborious effort. Many of the difficulties involved are those common to all pupils in reading, but are greatly accentuated.

Fernald (1943) calls them "cases of partial disability." She feels that "these cases usually develop normal reading skills when they are given the opportunity to learn by ordinary methods after the faulty conditions (poor vision or hearing, illness, emotional instability or lack of adequate schooling) have been removed." Vernon (1957) classifies this group as "backward readers" or "semi-illiterates." Johnson[1] states that a corrective case is "a case of reading retardation not complicated by neurological difficulties, deficiencies in associative learning, and so on." She feels that these cases may result from "lack of readiness when initial experiences with reading were provided, continued instruction above the proper level, lack of adequate stimulation in instruction, inadequate background of experience or oral language facility, and so on." The important thing is that these cases do not usually require clinical instruction unless the retardation is compounded by continued inattention to correction and attendant emotional complications.

Most corrective instruction is the responsibility of all teachers in their daily class activities. In some school systems a special reading teacher provides systematic instruction for small groups.

The procedure known as remedial reading, as contrasted with corrective reading, applies to a small clinical group showing severe symptoms of reading retardation. Children in this group differ from those in the corrective group by the degree of their deficiency. The

---

[1] Statements made in a speech by Dr. Marjorie Johnson, the acting director of the Reading Clinic at Temple University.

cases are frequently characterized by associative learning disability, inadequacies in memory span, deficiencies in concept formation, and neurological or emotional complications. Pupils with these problems demand individual and small-group instruction on a clinical basis by specially trained personnel. It is often in this last group that reading difficulty may result in real damage to the personality. A child who cannot read or who cannot read as well as his group is marked before everyone as a failure. He is reminded of failure many times a day and every day. Even a skilled classroom or corrective-reading teacher often cannot restore his confidence in himself since his classmates and scolding parents often magnify his deficiency.

Vernon (1957) labels these pupils "illiterates" and defines them as "those who for some reason or other are unable to master even the simpler mechanics of reading." Fernald (1943) calls their conditions "total or extreme disabilities." She defines these disabled readers as those "individuals who fail to learn to read under the most careful instruction by methods that are successful with the average child." Other educators classify this group as "word blind" or "alexic" or "dyslexic," while members of the Orton Society diagnose these cases as having a specific reading disability of the strephosymbolic type. Mrs. Orton (1957) pointed out some of the following characteristics:

1. They show no evidence of any significant impairment of vision or hearing, or brain damage, or primary personality deviations, or any history thereof.

2. They show great difficulty in remembering whole-word patterns, and do not learn easily by the "sight method."

3. They are poor oral readers and fundamentally poor spellers.

4. They usually come from families in which there is left-handedness or language disorders, or both.

5. In their early attempts at reading and writing, they show marked confusions in remembering the orientation of letters (b, d, p, q) and the order of letters in words or numbers in

sequences (was-saw, on-no, felt-left, 12-21). They are sometimes called "mirror-minded" or "mirror-readers."

6. They usually show some evidence of delayed or incomplete establishment of one-sided motor preferences. They tend to be left-handed or ambidextrous, or mixed in their motor choices, e.g., right-handed and left-eyed, or they may have been slow in the establishment of their handedness.

7. They often show delays or defects in more than one language area. In addition to poor reading, they may have delayed or imperfect speech; a poor ear for words; a poor oral vocabulary; or clumsiness in handwriting or in other motor acts.

Gallagher (1960) summarizes the Orton outlook as follows:

> Specific language disability has also been termed specific reading disability, congenital dyslexia, congenital word blindness, etc., and is one of the many causes of scholastic failure. When present, it is a handicap to a pupil, even though failure may not result. Its basic cause, though still unknown, would seem to be a disturbance in neurological function, but it should be distinguished from neurological disorders which are less amenable to treatment—such as those from intellectual and sensory deficits, and from learning problems primarily due to emotional disturbances.

Educators for a number of years have had effective developmental and corrective reading programs in the public schools. Developmental programs usually run from grades one through six (although many school systems now have programs in grades seven and eight), and corrective programs are established in local elementary and secondary schools throughout the country.

In most school systems a lack of funds, trained personnel, or a general unawareness of the problem have prevented the development of a clinically oriented program for the remedial-illiterate-wordblind-strephosymbolic-totally-disabled reader.

Surveys of the literature reveal the disturbing fact that educators, even when they recognize the problem, often cannot agree on a name for these pupils—let alone their symptoms or methods of remedying their condition.

In fact, even in the school systems that are involved in this area, we find most of the research being conducted by special education departments in a search for new pedagogical techniques for the brain-damaged and aphasic child.

In addition to this confusion, researchers have been searching for a common syndrome. A typical formula appears to call for administering a series of tests to a matched group of retarded and achieving readers. Statistical analysis such as the "T" test or analysis of variance is then applied to check the null hypothesis. Whenever the variable is statistically significant, or the null hypothesis rejected, another part of a syndrome is developed. We all are aware of the importance and weakness of statistics in dealing with the human organism—the situation, size and composition of the sample, and bias of the experimenters have in fact resulted in a great deal of confusion about these cases in the literature of reading retardation. Helen Robinson (1946) only used 30 retarded readers for her classic text, *Why Pupils Fail in Reading*. Delacato (1959) analyzed 45 boys who were poor readers. Smith and Carrigan (1959) looked at 40 elementary students in their original testing program. Many other researchers have conscientiously conducted similar research and overestimated their success in marking out the total or partial answer to the problem. Instead of cooperative interdisciplinary studies, we have had a profusion of small cults, all proclaiming their discovery of the cure-all, the magic panacea. Pity the school teacher who tries to absorb and conscientiously practice the numerous "antidotes." Can anyone wonder why we are so confused?

Several years ago educators in the Baltimore County Public Schools decided to attempt to develop a remedial program. I should like to review here the results obtained during the 1960/1961 school year.

This remedial reading program is a clinical type of program designed for the retarded reader with an intelligence slightly below average, average, or superior, who cannot profit from the pedagogical techniques that are used in the regular developmental or corrective programs. The following criteria and procedures have been developed:

Who *should* be referred—

1) Students who have average, above average, or slightly below average intelligence and who exhibit difficulty with some or many phases of reading. These children combine an average or a high capacity level and a low achievement level. If they are read to, they are able to comprehend, and answer questions about, information beyond the level at which they read independently with understanding.

2) Students who seem to be intelligent enough to read at a much higher level than they do, even though their intelligence-test scores are a great deal below average.

This last is a very important point. McLaulin and Schiffman (1960) made a study of the relationship between the California Test of Mental Maturity and the WISC scores for retarded readers. Evidence was found that low scores obtained by children who have reading difficulties frequently reflect their degree of retardation rather than their basic capacity to learn. An examination of a sample of 60 clinically referred pupils who had been diagnosed as in need of remedial reading revealed a mean IQ score of 79 when measured by the CTMM. The same sample of pupils yielded a mean IQ of 95 when measured by the WISC, indicating a mean IQ difference of 16 points. There is no question that when group intelligence tests are used, the IQs of children who have severe reading disabilities present an erroneous picture of the learning capacity of these children.

The following types of students *should not* be referred—

1) Mentally retarded or very slow-learning students who are reading as well as students with their mental capacity can be expected to read.

2) Students with average or superior intelligence who are not reading quite as well as they might, but the difference between their achievement and capacity is not significant enough to request outside help.

3) Students who have learning problems other than reading.

4) Students who are disciplinary problems because of factors other than deficiencies in reading.

Referral Procedures—

1) Referrals to the remedial reading clinic should come from the (*a*) corrective teachers or (*b*) psychologists.

2) The remedial reading clinician diagnoses the needs of the pupil and one of the following procedures is pursued: (*a*) The pupil is assigned to the remedial clinic where an individual program is planned by the clinician and the remedial teacher. (*b*) If the pupil is not found to be in need of remedial assistance, he is returned to either the corrective or developmental program. (*c*) If it is found that the pupil's problem is not primarily reading, he is referred to the proper service.

3) When it is determined that a child should be placed in the remedial reading program, the reading specialist contacts his parents to explain the nature of this service and secure permission for this placement. Parents are responsible for transporting the pupil to and from the clinic for instruction.

4) A pupil is dismissed from the remedial clinic when the reading specialist feels the pupil is ready to progress in either the corrective or the developmental program.

Proper diagnosis of reading problems and reading levels is made possible by the use of the following apparatus in a complete reading analysis: (*1*) social, familial, developmental, and school case histories; (*2*) individual intelligence or capacity test; (*3*) personality evaluation including the Rorschach and Draw-A-Person; (*4*) a reading battery including standardized achievement tests and informal reading skills analysis; (*5*) Gates Associative Learning Test; (*6*) Detroit Tests of Memory Span; (*7*) Laterality Tests to determine eye and hand dominance; (*8*) physical screening; (*9*) Bender Visual-Motor Gestalt Test; (*10*) Frostig Perceptual Development Examination; (*11*) Eisenson Examination for Aphasia.

An explanation of some of these tests may help in understanding this important step in the reading program.

General intelligence or capacity. The individual intelligence test such as the Wechsler or the Binet is given rather than a standardized paper-pencil test which depends on the child's reading ability. It should be pointed out that some pupils might have difficulty concentrating or in doing those sections of the test which are similar to academic situations. For this reason the performance score might be a higher and more accurate indication of the child's true potential than the verbal score.

Altus (1956), Kallos, Grabow and Guarino (1961) and others indicate that an analysis of the individual WISC pattern may have diagnostic value for predicting reading disability. Many researchers feel that a statistically low coding and arithmetic score correlates highly with severe reading disabilities. Our research with over four hundred clinically referred remedial readers seems to agree with these findings.

Two informal measures that have particular diagnostic value are the Word Recognition Test and the Informal Reading Inventory.

Word Recognition Test. This test is made up of word lists consisting of fifteen to twenty-five words at each level—preprimer through tenth grade. The words themselves are based on word frequency counts of books commonly used in grades one through ten.

The test is designed to determine the student's word recognition ability at various grade levels and to diagnose specific word perception needs. The test has two parts: the flash section which enables one to determine the sight vocabulary of the pupil; and the untimed section which reveals the pupil's ability to employ word-attack skills. In administering the test each word is presented for approximately one second. If the word is pronounced correctly, the teacher continues down the list. If a word is mispronounced it is exposed again for as long as the student may require. (This untimed exposure reveals his word-attack skills.) Comprehension cannot be tested by this device. True remedial cases usually have considerable difficulty with this test; some corrective cases may also have difficulty, but the latter may have only comprehension problems.

Informal Reading Inventory (IRI). This is the principal instrument in discovering the specific reading needs of the reader. It consists of two selections from each graded basal reader—preprimer through the ninth grade. Usually the informal inventory is started one grade below the level at which the first error was made on the word recognition flash test.

In administering this test the teacher first has the student set up a purpose for reading. The student then reads orally and the teacher asks questions (factual, vocabulary, and critical) concerning the material. These steps are repeated in connection with another, and silent, reading. As a result the teacher gets information about the student's reading levels and his needs.

Usually auditory and visual discrimination tests are administered. Even at the secondary level severely retarded pupils have trouble with basic auditory and visual discrimination skills that the average six-year-old child taking his reading readiness test could easily pass.

I hesitate to list symptoms but some of the obvious findings that contribute to the diagnosis of a clinically retarded reader are:

1) Low frustration level in word recognition abilities, with a sight vocabulary inadequate at a low level and very few word analysis skills evident at any level.

2) No improvement in oral rereading.

3) In the capacity measures, the child scores higher in the non-verbal than in the verbal tests. Also its performance in subtests involving memory association, organization, and persistence is limited.

4) In the associative learning tests the demands on visual-auditory abilities are greater than on visual-visual abilities and the geometric patterns are greater than the wordlike patterns.

5) In the memory span tests the forward span of digits is greater than the reversed span, the span for oral directions is usually very low, and the span for visual objects is greater than the span for visual letters.

After the pupil has been classified as in need of remedial treatment by the reading specialist, the psychologist and the reading clinician meet to select the students who can profit most by this type of program. The program is so geared that one reading center covers a wide area and only a small percentage of the candidates can be accepted. (We find in this candidate group from one to nine per cent of our school registration.) If the child is accepted, the parents are notified of their responsibilities to the program. They must provide transportation to the reading clinic each day, and attend PTA and Parent Life Discussion Group meetings. The elementary-school child reports to the building at 9:00 o'clock each morning and is picked up by the parent at 11:40 and taken to the regular school for the afternoon session. The parents of the second-ary-school child must also provide transportation. The student is picked up at his regular school each day and transported to the clinic by 12:45 P.M. Classes are dismissed at 3:30 P.M. and parents make arrangements to call for their child at that time.

Seven PTA meetings are scheduled during the school year. Three meetings are conducted by the reading clinician who leads a highly structured meeting. The other four meetings are headed by a visit-ing teacher trained in Family Life Discussions. The parents have an opportunity to discuss some of the things, either old or new, that have been bothering them. Here the parents see that they are not alone; other parents have similar problems; other children have personality difficulties. In many cases parents can help each other solve some of these pressing issues. The whole program is con-ducted in a nondirective, relaxed fashion and acts as a kind of catharsis. The psychologist and reading clinician are there as ob-servers, and only join in as consultants when requested by the parents. The group discusses such practical problems as: How do I make my child do his homework? How should I handle my child now that he is so aggressive? Family Life meetings assume that all children who need the remedial reading program are emotionally disturbed to some degree. Therefore, it is felt that therapy for the children and discussion groups for the parents should be an integral part of the program. The aim is to develop and increase parental understanding of the emotional growth and emotional needs of the children. Here are some of the parents' comments concerning last year's meetings:

> We feel that it has helped to be associated with people who have similar problems.
> We now feel better prepared to handle the problems we now have and also feel more confident about facing the problems that may be ahead of us.
> Please accept our appreciation for the understanding we have devel-oped.

As far as the educators were concerned, they felt that the discus-sion groups were of great benefit. Parents relaxed and felt free to discuss their anxieties openly after the first session. The greatest value came to the parents through their own interchange of experiences. Parents' insight seemed to be improved. Children were benefited by the improved attitude of the parents.

Now let us look at the actual program in the clinic. As stated before, elementary-school students attend in the morning; secondary-school students in the afternoon. Whenever possible, the programs are so structured in the local school that the youngsters attend classes and participate in activities requiring limited reading and writing skills. This, of course, is much easier to do in the secondary program. However, we have found in the fourth, fifth, and sixth grades where reading is conducted in the morning that the pupils can meet success in the afternoon in some subjects that do not depend directly on the children's reading ability. Ideally, the reading specialist works with about seven youngsters in each morning and afternoon session.

Grouping as far as instruction is concerned is very fluid. It varies with the immediate needs of the individual. The pedagogical program still centers around the Directed Reading Activity (we use our own basal readers, the Chatto and Windus series, and rewritten material), and the experience approach. This latter psychological approach utilizes the tracing or VAKT[2] techniques instead of simply the VA techniques that are used in the developmental and corrective programs. Evidence is leading us to believe that certain severe disabilities are alleviated through the use of a synthetic or Gillingham approach. Fernald tracing techniques have also been valuable. Also, some selected pupils may obtain help in developing hand and eye coordination and visual perceptual skills.

The important thing to remember is that there is no one approach to remediate these severely retarded readers. Three techniques should be considered:

1) The basal or experience approach using V and A.

2) The Fernald approach using VAKT in analytical breakdown.

3) The Gillingham approach using VAKT in a synthetic method.

Orton (1957) has summarized all of the approaches in two basic principles:

[2] Visual, Auditory, Kinesthetic, Tactile

1) Start the language training with small units which the pupil can handle easily and then proceed by orderly steps from the simple to the more complex. Be sure to teach the blending of the separate units into meaningful wholes. This approach can be applied to speech, handwriting, and motor skills as well as to reading and spelling.

2) Use all sensory pathways to reinforce the weak memory patterns and to strengthen one another. For example, have the pupil look at the letter, hear or say its sound, and trace it simultaneously. Or later, in working on comprehension, have him try to get the main idea of a paragraph from hearing it read aloud, reading it aloud, reading it silently, and expressing his ideas either orally or in writing. Comprehension can be improved upon occasion by drawing or making models from written directions. Combine the eye, the ear, and the hand—and always work toward the over-all grasp of meaning.

The program is so geared that the youngsters have a wide variety of high-interest, low-reading-level material supplemented by such kits and gadgets as tape recorders, filmstrips, slide projectors, hand and eye coordinators, primer typewriters, and SRA[3] material. During the day, a certain number of youngsters will visit with the psychologists for individual and group therapy. There is no apparent direct relationship between the psychologist and the reading teacher. Each never invades the other's domain. The children cannot play one against the other. They soon realize that there is no stigma attached to being in the program; everyone in the clinic has a reading problem; everyone has an opportunity to meet success at his proper instructional level.

Here is a report of a play session that Mr. Roger Saunders had with three of the elementary pupils.

> Bill and John quickly started playing together with the Tinker Toys but, when both wanted to build a proper foundation, they could not agree as to which foundation would be best; consequently, Bill gave up fairly quickly and began to play with Jane. This did not last too long and Bill went back to building something of his own, but this time

[3] Science Research Associates, Inc., Chicago 11, Ill., distributors of materials of instruction, tests, etc.

without competing with John. (Perhaps this shows us something about Bill's ability to tolerate competition.) Later Jane, who had not played with Tinker Toys before, was not doing anything and I suggested that she might be interested in building something, to which she reacted in a negative way. With slight pressure she chose to build a telescope tower. I helped her and we did complete this task. By the end of the task, Bill had given up his game and was helping and wanted to finish it with his imagination rather than sticking to the rules. I demanded attention to the rules, and in a fairly pleasant way the thing was finished. He felt that he could see Bridget Bardot and Marilyn Monroe through the telescope, and we all laughed at that. John continued to work alone creating an elaborate and impractical design. When these tasks were finished, the boys began to wrestle and John quickly got Bill down and held him down until I interrupted for cleanup time.

The afternoon program is structured almost the same as this. However, the youngsters in the afternoon program, being somewhat more mature, have individual therapy sessions instead of play therapy. They also work independently more than the morning youngsters.

The actual value of therapy in conjunction with remedial assistance is still under question. The research that has been published so far is quite controversial and varied. Arthur (1940) gave a number of examples of children with severe reading problems who were helped with psychiatric treatment, enabling them to improve their reading levels. Axline (1947) and Lecky (1945) have postulated that poor reading may result from inconsistencies in the attitudinal system of a child, or from difficulty in resolving a conflict between a concept of self as a poor reader and a concept of self as a good reader. A study by Bills (1950), using nondirective play therapy with a group of retarded readers, suggests that significant gains in reading may be accomplished by therapy alone.

A recent study (1961) conducted in Baltimore County investigated the value of remedial reading with psychotherapy in the public-school system. A sample of forty students was selected and randomly divided into four equal groups. One group received remedial reading and psychotherapy; one group received remedial reading only; one group received psychotherapy only; the fourth group received no treatment. See, Joss, Leiman, and Schiffman.

Using a gain in reading grade-level as a criterion, and removing initial differences between treatment groups by analysis of covariance, hypotheses were tested as to the effect of the four methods on reading ability.

The experiment showed a positive effect in favor of remedial reading as a treatment; yet shows no consistent effect due to psychotherapy. This study was conducted with such a small sample that we feel psychotherapy nevertheless cannot be ignored as a clinical procedure with retarded readers. It appears necessary to gather more evidence before making a decision in this matter. This study will be replicated on a much larger scale during the next two years.

The reading teachers in our program have constant conferences either by telephone, letter, or in person with the classroom teacher to integrate and correlate the two programs. The reading teachers also meet with the psychologists to discuss how the youngsters are progressing in the program. Once a month, the entire staff meets in an evaluation program. Whenever the student is academically and psychologically prepared, he is returned to the corrective or the developmental program. If the youngster is not meeting any success, he may be returned to the local school for further study and recommendations. The program has developed to such an extent that we have four remedial centers this year. Next year we will add at least one more center so that we will be able to cover Baltimore County effectively, and the pupils will not have to travel so far to take advantage of these programs.

A study of the results of the last three academic years of the entire program is quite extensive since there were over six thousand pupils in the corrective reading program and one hundred pupils in the remedial.

Tables 1 and 2 give data that seem significant as far as the corrective program is concerned.

Table 1. Reading Growth of Elementary and Secondary School Pupils Receiving Corrective Instruction During 1960/61 Year.

Years Growth in Reading	-.49-.00	.00-.49	.50-.99	1.00-1.49	1.50-1.99	2.00-2.49	2.50-2.99	3.00-3.49	3.50-3.99	4.00-4.49	4.50-4.99	5.00-5.49	Total
Number of Elementary Pupils	37	96	215	224	371	173	56	29	34	—	—	—	1235
Number of Secondary Pupils	6	60	110	228	92	270	100	141	15	36	2	16	1076
Total Number of Pupils	43	156	325	452	463	443	156	170	49	36	2	16	2311

Summary of results:
1) Average growth in years for elementary pupils: 1.5 years.
2) Average growth in years for secondary pupils: 2.0 years.
3) Average growth in years for all pupils: 1.75 years.

It appears quite obvious that the most success in remediating the reading problem is obtained in the early lower grades. If we could concentrate our efforts in the primary grades, we could return more pupils more quickly to their regular developmental program. The only reason I mention this here is because I believe that early diagnosis and remediation is so necessary.

Table 2. Percentages of Corrective Reading Pupils Reading at Their Proper Level at End of 1960/61 Year.

Grades	2	3	4	5	6	7	8	9
Extraclassroom corrective instruction received	82	46	42	18	8	10	11	6
Extraclassroom corrective instruction not received	18	6	6	3	1	.5	.25	.25

The academic results obtained in the three remedial clinics during the 1960/61 year are summarized in the following table:

Table 3.   Summary of Results

	Number of Students			Average Growth in Reading		
	Elementary	Secondary	Total	Elementary	Secondary	Average
Clinic I	10	9	19	2.03	2.78	2.41
Clinic II	11	8	19	2.27	3.19	2.73
Clinic III	8	9	17	2.94	3.11	3.02
Total/Average	29	26	55	2.41	3.03	2.72

In summary, I would like to say that I do not believe that any one discipline—whether medical or educational—or any one technique will by itself solve this serious problem. No one discipline will be able to answer these questions: What is the etiology of these disabilities? How can we make an early diagnosis? What are the best pedagogical procedures in remediating these specific language disabilities?

Clemmens (1961) discusses this problem in his paper, *Minimal Brain Damage in Children, an Interdisciplinary Problem: Medical, Para-Medical and Educational.* The title of his paper "denotes those professional areas which are concerned with these children and connotes the possible imperfect understanding of the problem by these professions." He makes one observation that is so significant: "In an age of specialization we have not cultivated the inter-professional communications and exchange of ideas which are necessary for our mutual understanding of these complex problems." But an interdisciplinary approach, investigating and refining diagnostic and pedagogical techniques, is the only logical attack.

If we constantly re-evaluate and improve what we have, some day we will find what we need—a program to rehabilitate these lost children and give every child in our schools an opportunity to develop his language abilities to the highest level of his capacity.

4

A Study of Reading Achievement in a Population of School Children

J. R. NEWBROUGH AND
JAMES G. KELLY

This paper[1] will discuss a research program which approaches the topic of this conference rather differently than the other papers. The major difference is that our attention has been directed to the study of the entire range of reading achievement in a large group of school children. We will present (*1*) some of the problem areas in methodology which have been of concern to us, and (*2*) the process of an epidemiological study; both of which illustrate how population research differs from clinical research.

Population research provides a means by which a group of similar individuals (e.g., school children) are selected. Subgroups displaying the presence or absence of a condition (e.g., reading disability) are specified and their identifying characteristics (e.g., age, sex, IQ, social status) are determined. The central question in *population studies* would be something like "How many cases of reading disability exist in this group and how are they different from at-grade

[1] We are indebted to our assistants, Mae E. Rosenberg, Stephen Kappel, Elaine Carnvale, Natalie Bates, and to our consultant in epidemiology, Raymond Seltser, for their helpful comments and criticisms.

or advanced readers?" In *case studies* a major concern could be described as, "What specifically is characteristic of these individuals who display poor reading achievement?" With both approaches, one obtains a broader range of knowledge about the nature of reading achievement. As an example of considering this problem in many ways, the participants at this symposium are concerned with dyslexia as (*1*) a neurologically based phenomenon; (*2*) a perceptual difficulty; (*3*) a dysfunction of cognitive integration; (*4*) a complex condition to be classified in several ways so that appropriate educational measures can be taken; and (*5*) a condition which exists in a school population and which may be associated with poor adjustment. These approaches complement each other and should result in a more complete understanding of the condition *reading disability.*

The Epidemiological Study of Reading Achievement: An Example

This project, entitled Reading Ability and Outcome, is an example of epidemiological methods applied to the study of reading achievement in a population of 4080 sixth-grade school children. The project is being carried out in the Community Projects Section of the Mental Health Study Center, Langley Park, Maryland. It involves all 85 public schools of a county.

Epidemiology refers to an approach, developed in public health, to determine the extent and characteristics of a disease within population groups. Its early applications were in the study and control of epidemics which were so frequent and widespread in the eighteenth and nineteenth centuries (Kappel and Bates [1961]; Rosen [1958]). The method involves counting cases in the group under study and determining the identifying characteristics of the condition. Records are often the main source of data since they provide readily accessible sources of information on a large number of individuals. As the record-keeping improves, so does the precision and accuracy of the results of these studies. As epidemiological procedures have become more refined, data have been made available through special collections, such as surveys. Most epidemiological research, however, continues to be based on some record-keeping procedure.

This study is an example of records research. Achievement and adjustment information is collected on each student in school. We chose to use the classroom testing reports and the cumulative record cards as primary data sources. The study was designed to elucidate the characteristics of differing levels of readers (defined by the California Achievement Test)[2] and to follow them over a six-year period. The follow-up study is to provide information on the eventual academic and social adjustment of the children who were identified as retarded, normal-for-grade, and advanced readers.

Methodological Problems

Sampling, measurement of the reading level, and definition of retardation presented us with some difficult problems.

Sampling. Population studies include in their scope the whole range of the condition under scrutiny; for example, we study normal and high reading performances as well as the low. For this reason we select the subjects for our study on a criterion different from the matter under study (in this case, reading achievement) (Mac-Mahon, Pugh, and Ipsen [1960]). To measure reading achievement we would have to select a large group of children of a specific age, grade, or locality and determine the reading characteristics of the entire group. This technique differs from that of the clinical study which selects subjects because they exhibit the disability. The subjects for clinical study are selected as representative of the disabled

---

[2] The California Achievement Test is a minor revision of the Progressive Achievement Test, 1943 revision. There are ten subtests covering reading, arithmetic, and language skills. Comprehension and vocabulary are the reading skills which are measured and included in the Reading Section Score. A detailed description is provided by Buros (1953; 1959) and California Test Bureau (1957).

readers; the subjects for population study, as representative of the entire group of readers.

The population chosen for our study comprised all students who were enrolled in the regular sixth-grade classes in the county in 1954/55, and who had been administered standard achievement tests. Miller, Margolin, and Yolles (1957), the early investigators for this project, reasoned that all of the students in any particular grade in the public-school system should provide a representation of the county's school-age children.

Data collection on a population often affects the sampling. After the subjects have been selected, one must contend with such problems as refusals to cooperate, absences from home, changes of interviewers, and the like (Goldfarb [1960]). Our use of school records presented some of these problems. Since we identified the children by reading scores, we were faced with the fact that over a hundred children were absent from school on the testing day and thus were not tested. For a small number of other children, we were unable to locate their school progress cards, although the classroom testing records are available. This means that within each group the total number of responses will vary slightly; it means, too, that the data represent a somewhat smaller number of subjects than are in the population group.

The major difficulty in longitudinal studies is the loss of sample or withdrawal from the population group. This is the bane of longitudinal research because the loss of individuals can markedly change the composition and representation of the subject group. To illustrate how representation changes: slightly over half of our population group did not graduate from the high schools in the county in June, 1961, that is, when the sixth-graders of 1954/55 were due to graduate. This means that the remainder fell behind their class, transferred out of the county, or dropped out of school. An analysis of the reading scores of the children we are as yet unable to locate shows that (using the definition of plus or minus two grade years) seventeen per cent were retarded and three per cent were advanced (see Table 1, p. 72). This compares with fourteen per cent retarded and five per cent advanced among the entire population. Further follow-up study is needed to determine whether or not these unlocated subjects will eventually fall more frequently into the retarded group. We have hypothesized that this should happen for those who dropped out of school.

Measurement of reading level. Reading performance of this group of school children was measured by the California Achievement Test. Separate scores for Reading Vocabulary and Reading Comprehension are combined for a Reading Section score. This approach contrasts with clinical studies which use batteries of individual tests such as the Gates Reading Diagnosis Tests or the Gray Standardized Oral Reading Paragraphs, not only to assess reading achievement, but to diagnose the various skills involved in reading (Harris and Roswell [1953]). These tests are much more specialized than the group tests, and are regarded as more precise—much as the individual intelligence test is preferred to a group test like the California Test of Mental Maturity.[3]

Group tests for assessment of abilities have a history dating from the First World War when it was necessary to screen large numbers of recruits. Since that time the tests have become more refined and increasingly precise and accurate in their assessment of performance (Nunnally [1959]). Judging from its standardization and from the review literature, it appears that the California Achievement Test is widely used and correlates rather well with other achievement tests (Buros [1953]; California Test Bureau [1957]; Traxler and Jungeblut [1960]; Traxler and Townsend [1955]).

In the design of this study, reading scores were hypothesized to be predictors of later outcomes; for example, low reading scores in the sixth grade may be the basis for the prediction of specific kinds of social maladjustment in high school. Nunnally (1959) points out that a test which gives an accurate assessment of an ability (such as

---

[3] Individual tests of reading ability attempt to measure many more aspects of the process than do group tests, and they go much more into detail for each aspect than is possible on a group achievement test. In the case of the California Achievement Test, reading is one of three abilities measured; comprehension and vocabulary skills having been chosen as the more important for assessment. The Gates Reading Diagnosis Tests, on the other hand, provide twenty-one separate scores to describe the reading process; rate, size of vocabulary, retention and recognition of words, and errors in reading are examples of some of the scores.

reading) may not provide an accurate prediction of future behavior (such as social adjustment). He holds that assessment is the necessary prelude to prediction, and that occasionally tests designed for assessment purposes will also be predictive. It is, therefore, necessary to study whether the California Achievement Test can serve both an assessment and a prediction function.

Other problems in the measurement of reading level are the two elements often described as reliability and validity. Reliability, or consistency, refers to the degree to which the test measures the same things upon repeated application (American Psychological Association [1954]; Nunnally [1959]). Our group was tested for reading in the sixth, seventh, ninth, and eleventh grades. While this involved three different tests, it was first thought that this could provide an indication of the reliability of the measures. Since, however, the testings were at least one year apart, and more frequently separated by two years, it appeared that the individuals had sufficient time to show behavior changes that would not necessarily reflect the precision of the test. On the basis of this assumption, we decided to use already published literature to furnish information on reliability; the repeated testings will be used to assess the stability of the reading achievement of the subjects themselves over a five-year period.

Validity, or accuracy, indicates the degree to which the test measures what it purports to (American Psychological Association [1954]; Cronbach and Meehl [1955]; Ebel [1961]; Nunnally [1959]). Validity is ascertained by relating the scores of one test to another (called the criterion) which is known to measure the characteristic in question. With achievement tests, the usual practice is to relate a test to other achievement tests of accepted merit.[4]

We became interested in the validity problem when one of our assistants, in a review paper, indicated that there is some evidence that group achievement tests measure the reading level to be higher

---

[4] There will be possible a very rough validity check on the test results. The course grades assigned by the teacher can be compared to the level assigned by the achievement test to see how much agreement there is between the test and the teacher.

than do the individual tests (Rosenberg [1961]).[5] This might imply that the differences are due to errors in measurement. While such may be the case, Johnson (1961) provides a thesis which says, in effect, that the individual and group tests measure *different* things. She describes three levels of reading, each higher than the next; the *functional* level where the child reads independently, the *instructional* level where the child reads in the classroom, and the *frustrational* level, at which the student misses over half the material that he reads. It is her judgment that group tests measure the frustrational level, while individual tests can measure all three levels. It may make little difference, however, what reading level is being measured when one uses achievement test scores as predictors of later behavior. But the problem of accuracy does make difficult the evaluation of the results of assessment of *reading* achievement, and the comparison of results with other investigators who use different tests of reading ability.

Certainly the population researcher, using group tests, will get different results than someone using the clinical method. Effective communication becomes possible in such instances as this symposium when each can discuss what he is measuring, and each can try to determine how the tools relate to each other.

Definition of retardation. One of the most challenging problems in reading research is the definition and relative meaning of reading retardation. Our recent searches of the literature have failed to disclose any very comprehensive discussions of the concept. Several of the papers of this symposium have referred to the problem. We would like to see some discussion directed toward the formulation of an approach to the solution of this problem.

The definition of retardation has varied from one and one half to two grade level years of deviation from some standard of expected performance (either actual grade placement or mental age). Rabinovitch and co-workers (1954) used two years as their definition; this was also selected by Miller, Margolin, and Yolles (1957) for our early work with the sixth grade. This appears to be a point at

[5] The discrepancy ranges from one to four grade-equivalent years (Lewis [1961]).

which there is little disagreement about retardation being present. While such a conservative definition is useful in determining clinical cases, it presents problems for the population investigator. Such a standard may serve to provide a clearly defined group of retarded readers, but how then does one handle the readers who are not quite that retarded? Are they to be called normal readers? If they are, will not their data change the picture of what constitutes a normal reader? The same point holds for advanced readers. We may be in the position of having clearly defined extremes and a poorly defined middle group if we are to use three categories: retarded, normal, and advanced. This underscores the point that reading achievement, whether retarded or advanced, is *not* a unitary phenomenon, but an ability with many levels of proficiency.

The way we have chosen to deal with the apparent dilemma is purely an empirical one. We are allowing the actual reading scores to determine the distribution. This does not commit us prematurely to any definition of retardation and allows us to use successive grouping or statistical techniques to determine the dividing lines between different reading level groups. We can try out a number of definitions to see which best fits the data. Whatever dividing lines are selected, it seems now clear that three categories are not sufficiently descriptive of the nature of reading. Our thought runs to five, such as: retarded, slightly retarded, normal, slightly advanced, advanced. This represents one value of a population study; that is, the selection of a sufficient range of reading ability scores can help to define what differing reading levels mean.

Background and Method

So far we have described the issues which have concerned us in thinking about how the study should be carried out. We would like now to give a picture of the early phases of the study's development, and the current state of progress.

Over the past nine years there has been a developing interest at the Study Center in the subject of reading ability as it relates to mental health problems. Miller, Margolin, and Yolles (1957) described this interest and how it led to the present research. A study of the case files at the Study Center for the period 1948 to 1954 was made. Of the 427 children seen clinically for nonreading problems, a third of the boys and a fifth of the girls were retarded readers. In order to obtain perspective on the representative nature of these findings and to test some hypothesized outcomes, this population study was undertaken.

The study has had two time orientations: (1) the cross-sectional and (2) the longitudinal.

Cross-sectional approach. This study involves only the sixth-grade (1954/1955) data and is designed to provide a descriptive account of the population group at the beginning of the study. The analysis will follow two phases: descriptive and correlational.

The descriptive phase will provide tabulations of all the variables for the entire group, subdivided:

  a) as to school—85 different schools;
  b) as to sex—male, female;
  c) as to reading level—high, medium, low.

Beyond these tabulations, each of the variables (there are a total of 71) will be related to the others for the entire group as well as each of the subgroups defined by the sex, school, and reading-level characteristics. This will provide a picture of the interrelationships of such things as socio-economic status and extracurricular participation by each of the major groupings (sex, school, reading level).

The 85 schools serve as the major geographic units in the project. For each geographic area, such things as age, sex, and social class will be determined. Each school will be described by an average reading score, as well as the variability of reading scores. This approach is important in understanding the school environment to which children are exposed. It may help to explain why more poor readers occur in one school than in another. To illustrate, when the proportions of boys and girls retarded in reading by two or more years were plotted on the county map, in all districts save one there were more boys retarded. It would be of particular interest to determine why this one school had more retarded girls. For instance, are there more girls in this district, or is there some factor which affects girls only?

The tabulations and correlations will provide a series of descriptions of the population group. The analysis is expected to provide information which will help structure the hypotheses for the longitudinal phase. For example, knowing that low reading levels tend to be associated with boys, we will want to follow this characteristic over six years to see whether the relationships remain the same. The following questions are illustrative of those to be asked in the cross-sectional analysis.

1) How many children are retarded in reading in this group?

2) What characterizes the schools which have many low-scoring readers, as contrasted with schools which do not?

3) What other information on the record card is related to low reading achievement?

Longitudinal approach. The longitudinal method in epidemiology involves the selection of a large group or population to be followed for a specified time period. The group is followed to study outcomes. In this project the persons in the population identified as a risk group are the retarded readers. It is with these subjects that the undesirable outcomes (such as the leaving of school, or being referred to a social agency) will be expected. The rest of the population provides comparison groups to show whether any outcome is specific to one or general to all groups.

The major difficulty of population studies, as mentioned before, is the large number of persons who must be followed to obtain an adequate number of specific cases. In the study of low-scoring readers, the problem is not so acute since the definition of two years or more retarded applied to fully fourteen per cent of the population. The difficulty is likely to occur in the longitudinal phase where it will be necessary to determine and group the various eventual outcomes. Here sample size will be more of a problem.

Follow-up study has constituted the area of major effort so far. Two months' work has specifically accounted for over two thirds of the group. This leaves 1231 individuals yet to be specifically located at the point in time when they withdrew from school, were retained to repeat a grade, and so forth. Since somewhat less than half of the original group remained in the county school system to graduate, we must now try to determine what happened to the remainder, and how much longitudinal information is available. Ideally, we would like to trace the history of every member of the population, but this would be an expensive effort.

The following questions illustrate those to be asked in the longitudinal phase of this population study:

1) How stable are reading levels over a five-year period (measured at sixth, seventh, ninth, and eleventh grades)?

2) What proportion of low-scoring readers drop out of school, rather than merely transfer? Is there any relationship between the level of retardation and the time they drop out?

3) What are the academic experiences of the low-scoring readers who remain in school?

4) Do low-scoring readers and their families have more contact with social agencies than others in the group?

5) What outcomes are characteristic of the normal and high-scoring readers?

The longitudinal phase will be generally less descriptive than the earlier phase and will be aimed at answering specific questions or testing particular hypotheses. It is probably the method of epidemiology most productive of detailed information about specific topics.

Conclusion

We have tried in this paper to provide an example of a population study of reading achievement. In so doing, the differences in approach to subject selection, hypotheses, and methods between population and clinical methods were discussed. This study, Reading Ability and Outcome, is illustrative of records research. It incorporates both the cross-sectional and the longitudinal approaches to give perspective on the nature and extent of reading ability levels in a county. Since it is clear that population and clinical methods do approach the study of reading rather differently, they may be said to complement each other. Integration of the knowledge should lead to effective prevention, control, and treatment programs.

Table 1.   Distributions of Sixth Grade Reading Scores on 3946 of the 4080 Subjects: An Example of Incidence and Prevalence.*

I
Prevalence of Low, At-Grade, and High Readers

	Low (4.1)	At-Grade (4.1-8.1)	High (8.1)	No Score	Total
Number of Cases	567	3050	209	120	3946
Percentage of Total	14	78	5	3	100

II
Incidence of Withdrawals from School Between Sixth and Seventh Grades

Number of Cases in Sixth Grade	567	3050	209	120	3946
Number of Withdrawals	14	71	4	6	95
Percentage of Withdrawals	2.5	2.4	1.9	5	2.4

* Preliminary tabulations of an incomplete representation of the population group. Prevalence refers to the number of cases within a group at any one point in time. Incidence refers to the frequency of a given occurrence over a particular time.

5

Dyslexia: Psychiatric Considerations

RALPH D. RABINOVITCH

Reading problems in children, regardless of their cause, are of necessity a major concern of child psychiatry. A significant percentage of children referred for psychiatric study because of adjustment or behavior difficulties are found to have a problem in reading. The incidence of reading deficits in children referred to Hawthorn Center is particularly high because of our known special research interests and the inclusion of a language clinic as part of our services. The language clinic was developed because of demonstrated dire need; it was impossible for us to study a good many of our referrals without these special services. Equally evident was the fact that psychiatric treatment, especially of inpatients, could not be effective without concomitant reading therapy for many of our boys. So often the school social worker or pediatrician refers the child with the hope, and even expectation, that the psychiatric clinic will find the learning problem to be due to an "emotional block" and that through the magic of psychotherapy, perhaps limited to a few interviews, the child will be "released" to learn adequately. Such unrealistic expectations have, unfortunately, been fostered in part by the attitude of some of our colleagues in child psychiatry and related fields who have been prone to overgeneralize dynamic formulations. The problem is far more complex; and the understanding of the large mass of reading problems which we see represents, I believe, one of the major current challenges to our field.

Even the most cursory review of an extensive number of cases we have seen over the past fifteen years indicates the need for differential diagnosis in relation to reading problems. The reading difficulty must first be seen as a symptom rather than a diagnostic entity in itself, just as we now view juvenile delinquency or mental retardation. Because of this we have used the broad term *reading retardation* to describe all cases in which there is a significant discrepancy between the mental age on performance tests and the level of reading achievement. We have suggested three major groupings that have emerged in our diagnostic studies:

1) Capacity to learn to read is intact but is utilized insufficiently for the child to achieve a reading level appropriate to his intelligence. The causative factor is exogenous, the child having a normal reading potential that has been impaired by negativism, anxiety, depression, emotional blocking, psychosis, limited schooling opportunity, or other external influence. We diagnose these as *secondary reading retardation*.

2) Capacity to learn to read is impaired by frank brain damage manifested by clear-cut neurological deficits. The picture is similar to the adult dyslexic syndromes long familiar to clinicians. Other definite aphasic difficulties are generally present. The case history usually reveals the cause of the brain injury, common agents being prenatal toxicity, birth trauma or anoxia, encephalitis, and head injury. These cases are diagnosed as *brain injury with reading retardation*.

3) Capacity to learn to read is impaired without definite brain damage being suggested in the case history or upon neurological examination. The defect is in the ability to deal with letters and words as symbols, with resultant diminished ability to integrate the meaningfulness of written material. The problem appears to reflect a basic disturbed pattern of neurological organization. Because the cause is biological or endogenous, these cases are diagnosed as *primary reading retardation*.

Because its usage has become so ambiguous, we have tended to avoid "dyslexia," but I presume that most workers would include our groups two and three under the term.

As you would expect, it is much more difficult to be certain into which group a particular case fits than it is to recognize that there are the three groups. Criteria for differential diagnosis are still uncertain and the problem is complicated by much overlap. On a theoretical basis we recognize that children with a primary disability will exhibit definite deficiencies in their basic reading techniques, that is in the reading process itself. Impairments may be seen, for example, in such factors as visual memory and association, auditory discrimination and association, and directionality. Capacity to use these basic processes is considered intact in secondary or psychologically determined retardation. The differentiation appears to be relatively certain in the extreme cases and in practice we tend to consider those children with gross reading incompetence as presenting the primary disability, while we are more inclined to view minimal retardations as secondary. Recognizing this, Lauretta Bender (1954; 1956a) has taken exception to the differentiation itself, expressing the view that all cases are due to a developmental lag, with the severity extending through a continuum from mildest to most severe. It is difficult indeed to disprove the validity of her view although she too describes many children whose reading deficiency is due to cultural deprivation alone.

In evaluating the child's reading situation, we are interested in relating it to total learning process including such factors as: (*1*) *General intelligence:* both verbal and performance areas, noting, especially, significant deviations from the mean on specific subtests. (*2*) *Specific capacities:* including vision, hearing, neurological integration, visual-motor functioning as reflected in such tests as the Bender-Gestalt and figure drawings, and particular areas of language functioning to which I will refer later. (*3*) *Developmental readiness:* about which we now think we know much less than we did when we started our work. (*4*) *Emotional freedom to learn:* which calls for careful psychiatric assessment. (*5*) *Motivation:* a problem of growing relevance in the large group of general underachievers currently referred. (6) *Opportunity for learning:* including earlier teaching methods used.

Despite the neatness of all our attempted theoretical formulations, I must confess that in practice our group not infrequently arrives at a diagnosis such as "secondary retardation with a touch of primary disability."

I know that the major interest of this symposium is in the group of cases with severe disability, our primary retardation group, and I should like to describe more fully our work with these. For some years now we have been working intensively with these patients, attempting both detailed diagnosis as well as remedial therapy on both an individual and small-group basis. Like so many other workers, we have been impressed with the presence of language and conceptual difficulties, beyond the reading problem. These become more evident in the day-by-day remedial sessions where response to specific techniques can be evaluated over a long period; much is learned too from recording spontaneous conversation of the children in groups.

We have attempted to present a concise functional description of the clinical pathology of the primary reading retardation syndrome by conceiving, diagrammatically, of the reading incompetence as the surface syndrome. From the surface to the core are successive layers of the more basic aspects of the pathology, thus:

reading retardation

reading process disturbance

broader language deficits

specific conceptual deficiency: orientation

body image confusion(?)

We would like to comment briefly on each of the suggested levels of disturbance, as a focus for discussion. While we recognize many "exceptional" cases, we are describing the common symptom pattern of the syndrome.

1) The *reading retardation* is usually severe and many of our patients, first seen in adolescence, have virtually no sight vocabulary and no phonic recognition. Arithmetical competence is usually also very low although it may be somewhat higher than the reading level. Spelling ability, as expected, is grossly impaired and this is reflected in the child's attempt at writing to dictation.

2) *Reading process disturbance:* We have noted earlier the frequency of gross visual-memory and association deficiencies, auditory association deficiencies, and directional confusion. Long-term work with the patients suggests a difficulty in using forms and sounds as symbols or inability to attach conceptual meaningfulness to the learning. For example, differences in vowel sounds are readily appreciated when presented orally, but the sounds cannot be translated into their letter symbols.

3) *Broader language deficits* are recognized in specific difficulty in name finding, imprecise articulation and primitive syntax. The child is usually more competent in offering simple definitions for words presented to him than in using the same words spontaneously in conversation.

4) *Specific conceptual deficiency in orientation* appears to underlie the other language inadequacies. The difficulty is in translating perceptions into symbols. Thus the child has no difficulty in appreciating which of two people is taller but he cannot define their heights in feet. Similarly he is well aware of the fact that school is out in the hot weather but he cannot define that season as summer. With a view to exploring further this basic conceptual problem, we have devised a Hawthorn Concepts Scale which we hope may serve as a diagnostic and prognostic device with young children. Drs. Langman, Ingram and Kauffman of our Hawthorn group are now completing standardization of the test which we think has major relevance to reading pathology.

5) *Body-image* problems have been much less clearly demonstrated. We have used Benton's discrimination and localization tests and other approaches with uncertain results. The children tend to show marked subjective reaction to the orientational dilemma. At present we feel a need for much more work in this whole area.

Regarding etiology, following the lead of other workers, we tend to view the symptom complex as representing a developmental discrepancy, often familial in origin, and expressing a parietal or parietal-occipital dysfunction. Acquired brain injury is suspected in some cases, but these are the exceptions.

Our present work involves the four disciplines: psychology, education, neurology, and psychiatry. We are completing work on the Hawthorn Concepts Scale. We are now in the fourth year of a longitudinal study of reading progress of classes of children in public schools. A large battery of tests has been given, starting in the first grade, and two groups have been isolated for detailed comparative investigation, those at the highest and at the lowest end of the reading scale. From this, we hope to develop prognostic indices. Our psychologists are attempting to define more precise differential diagnostic criteria from psychological test data. Although the studies are not complete, all the data tend to point at least in one direction. The problem does not seem to be one in perception per se, but rather in the translation of perceptions into meaningful symbols that can be used in reading and related language functions.

Finally, a word about the psychiatric implications of reading problems. It is evident that children with marked incompetence in an area so vital to their ego-attitude, and sometimes to their survival in today's world, will suffer inordinately. Often bright, perceptive, and sensitive, they tend to react successively with anger, guilt feelings, depression, and, finally, resignation, and compromise with their hopes and aspirations. Lauretta Bender has pointed out interesting parallels between children with severe reading disability and with schizophrenia. While the core problems are very different, the sense of uncertainty about their world may be common. The schizophrenic child, because of his poorly defined ego boundaries, has this uncertainty. The dyslexic child may be similarly perplexed and lost because of his inability to deal with symbols, the language of his world. The fact that he appears normal, and is so except in the one area of his deficiency compounds his problem.

For those children with a mild reading retardation secondary to emotional problems, psychotherapy is indicated. For those with the primary or dyslexic syndrome the need is for intensive, long-term remedial therapy. Our experience at Hawthorn indicates dramatically the need for early intervention, as close to the first-grade level as possible. Therapy must take into account the basic language and conceptual problems as well as the reading disability; initial work on orientational concepts may well be indicated before, or at least concomitant with, specific reading training.

A major tragedy in our work with these patients is our inability to do the whole job with them; even with the best help we have to offer, results are usually limited. If a child with a severe primary *Remedy* retardation ultimately reaches a fifth- or sixth-grade level of reading competence, we have done well. Hopefully, we can do better with earlier diagnosis and more specific treatment, based on careful diagnosis of each child's remedial need. Meanwhile special reading classes in the public schools are still desperately few, although the recent development of good programs in many parts of the country has been encouraging. There is a need too for an adjusted curriculum for many of these children, throughout the school years. Ways must be found to train these bright, potentially capable children through new techniques that rely minimally on literacy. Such planning presents a challenge as yet barely recognized.

6

Dyslexia in Relation to Form Perception and Directional Sense*

ARTHUR L. BENTON

The Clinical Picture of Acquired Dyslexia[1]

Impairment in oral and silent reading is a common feature of aphasic disorders. In most cases, it is reasonable to think of the observed reading disability as being one further aspect of a total syndrome of language disturbance which is reflected in all modes of comprehension and expression of symbolic material. In some patients with predominantly or exclusively expressive oral language deficit, oral reading may be severely impaired while the capacity for silent reading for meaning is relatively preserved. This profile of reading abilities may be considered to reflect the total pattern of language disorder in these patients, which is characterized by more

* The personal investigations cited in this paper were supported by a research grant (B-616) from the National Institute of Neurological Diseases and Blindness, United States Public Health Service.

[1] The term *dyslexia* is used here in a general sense to refer to all types and degrees of impairment in reading which are observed in patients with cerebral disease and not in any of the specific senses (e.g., partial disability, episodic disability, rapid fatigability) to be found in the older literature.

severe expressive than receptive deficit. The opposite pattern (i.e., retained capacity for oral reading with loss of the ability to grasp or retain the meaning of symbolic material) is also encountered, although much less frequently. This pattern can also be considered as a reflection of the primary nature of the total aphasic picture which is characterized by fluent expression but with loss of appreciation of the semantic values of received propositions.

Impairment in oral and silent reading is also commonly shown by patients with severe visuoperceptive deficit, as reflected in an agnosia for forms or objects. Here again it is reasonable to think of the reading disability in these patients as being simply another manifestation of their basic visuoperceptive deficit. The perception of letters and words requires a certain degree of visual discriminative capacity and it is easy to understand why a patient who cannot differentiate one geometric form from another would also fail to differentiate letters or words from each other.

However, in addition to these types of reading impairment which occur within a setting of either general language impairment or general visuoperceptive disability, more specific types of dyslexia, which are similar in some respects to developmental dyslexia, are also encountered. These specific types of dyslexia may occur in the absence of obvious oral language disability or, if they appear in association with some degree of oral language disability, they are so much more severe that they cannot reasonably be considered to be simply one further expression of the general disability. Similarly, they can occur in the absence of indications of gross visual perceptive impairment with respect to nonsymbolic stimuli. Whether they are actually independent of oral language or general visuoperceptive deficit is, as we shall see, an unsettled question. The point to be emphasized is that, whatever be their relationship to oral language and visuoperceptive functions, these specific dyslexias cannot be dismissed as being merely partial expressions of a more pervasive disability.

Acquired specific dyslexia is a common enough phenomenon. It may appear as the last residue of an aphasia in regression or it may be present from the very beginning as the only, or the most severe, form of language disability shown by a patient. In order to distinguish it from dyslexia which is quite obviously part of a pervasive aphasic disorder, specific dyslexia is often designated as *agnosic dyslexia*. The term is in some respects a rather unfortunate one. On the one hand, it suggests that this condition belongs in the same category as object- and form-agnosia, color agnosia and agnosia for faces. This is certainly an open question. On the other hand, it suggests that specific dyslexia is not a true language disorder and this question too remains to be clarified. Specific dyslexia is also called "pure" or "isolated" dyslexia, the implication being that it is essentially independent of more general language or visuoperceptive deficit. But it is precisely this implication which has been the major subject of controversy regarding dyslexia during the past fifty years. I have chosen the name "specific dyslexia" to refer to these conditions since it seems less extreme than "pure" or "isolated" and at the same time avoids the suggestive implications of "agnosic dyslexia." It should be clearly understood, however, that these dyslexias are "specific" only in the sense that they cannot be regarded as being partial expressions of either a general aphasia or a pervasive visual agnosia.

As is true of practically all the behavioral disturbances which are observed in patients with cerebral disease, specific dyslexia has been found to occur in association with a variety of sensory and behavioral deficits, among them being one or another type of impairment in writing and in arithmetical calculation, deficits in tactile reading, color agnosia, impairment in the perception of space and form, somatoperceptual deficits such as astereognosis, finger agnosia and right-left disorientation, and right homonymous hemianopia. The particular combinations of deficits which are observed vary from case to case. One dyslexic will show practically no disturbance in writing while another will show marked impairment in all aspects. A third may be able to write to oral dictation but not from written copy. The ability to recognize letters and numbers drawn on the skin surface and the capacity to profit from kinesthetic cues in reading vary widely from case to case. The association of dyslexia with defects in the naming and sorting of colors (so-called color agnosia) is observed in some cases. A right homonymous hemianopia is found in a majority of cases but not in all.

Thus, a great variety of individual clinical pictures is encountered. Beginning with Wernicke and Dejerine, students of dyslexia have sought to reduce this heterogeneity by classifying the disorder into types, each of which, it was hoped, would form a relatively consistent clinical picture. In general, two major types of acquired specific dyslexia have been described:

The first is so-called "parietal" dyslexia, which appears to be relatively independent of oral language disturbance but which is associated with severe dysgraphia, all aspects of writing being disturbed. Thus, it is actually a combined dyslexia-dysgraphia. And it is much more than that. Arithmetical calculation is likely to be impaired and drawing is almost invariably defective. Constructional tasks, such as stick-arranging and block-building, may be performed defectively. Orientation toward one's own body may be impaired. As its name implies, the responsible lesions in "parietal" dyslexia are presumed to be in the posterior parietal lobe, particularly in the regions of the angular and supramarginal gyri.

Thus, the dyslexia in these cases occurs against a background of generally disturbed spatial abilities, particularly as they are expressed in action. It is quite evidently part of a syndrome which is referable to parietal lobe disease and there is a great temptation to view it as simply one of several expressions of a basic disorder of spatial thinking in these patients. The idea is an attractive one and it may be correct. But there are considerations which militate against it. Unlike most other parietal deficits, dyslexia is specifically associated with disease of the left (i.e., dominant) hemisphere. If it were simply a partial expression of a more basic perceptual disability, it should appear in lesions of the right as well as of the left hemisphere. Indeed, considering the frequency with which visuospatial impairment is found in right hemisphere disease, one might well expect dyslexia to be a particularly prominent symptom; but it is not. There is the further fact that a patient may show relatively severe perceptual impairment as expressed in defective performance in writing, drawing, and constructional praxis tasks, and yet show no noteworthy dyslexia. It would seem then that, although the factor of perceptual impairment cannot be ignored, one must also invoke a specific linguistic or symbolic element to describe the condition adequately. An observation in consonance with this idea is that many of these patients, although not judged to be dysphasic by conventional clinical criteria, actually do show a higher-level semantic defect in their inadequate comprehension of complex propositions and their occasional word-finding difficulty. Thus, this type of dyslexia may be the resultant of a combination of perceptual and conceptual deficits (i.e., it may include both agnosic and aphasic components).

The second type of dyslexia is that which Dejerine called "word blindness with preservation of writing" and which Wernicke designated as "subcortical alexia." In contrast to the first type, it might be called "occipital" dyslexia. The patient with this impairment can write spontaneously and to dictation, although the writing will show minor imperfections. Writing that is copied from a model is likely to be quite poor. There are no obvious disturbances in oral language but difficulties in the naming, identification, and sorting of colors are frequent. A right homonymous hemianopia is almost invariably present. In contrast to the "parietal" type, the reading of the patient with "occipital" dyslexia may be significantly facilitated if he traces the letters or words, i.e., if kinesthetic cues are provided to aid perception. It has generally been thought that the responsible lesion involves the parieto-occipital area of the dominant hemisphere, particularly the basal parts of the occipital lobe and the angular gyrus. Geschwind, however, has adduced evidence that the crucial lesion must involve the splenium of the corpus callosum as well as the left occipital lobe.[2] Patients who have undergone left occipital lobectomy invariably show this type of dyslexia, either permanently or for some period of time.

"Occipital" dyslexia poses interpretive problems which are as difficult as those posed by "parietal" dyslexia. Many case reports describe the disability in an allegedly pure form. However, many clinicians have denied the reality of pure word blindness and insist that careful examination of these cases would disclose defects in the perception of nonsymbolic material as well as letters, words, and numbers.

[2] See below, p. 119.

There seems to be little doubt that they are right. Every case of specific dyslexia which has been studied in recent years, no matter how "pure" at first glance, has shown other types of perceptual, language, or motor impairment as well, e.g., some degree of visual form agnosia, impairment in the visual apprehension of relatively complex situations such as action pictures and cartoons, deficits in the recognition of colors, retardation in perceptual speed, impairment in memory, disordered eye movements in reading or higher-level defects in oral language. Yet, as is the case with "parietal" dyslexia, it is difficult to ascribe the dyslexia in any simple, direct way to these associated deficits since they vary from case to case, are often present to only a minor degree and are found in patients who are not dyslexic. Again the question is raised whether one must not think in terms of an interaction of perceptual and linguistic deficits to account for this form of specific dyslexia.

Acquired and Developmental Dyslexia Compared

There are obvious dissimilarities between acquired specific dyslexia and developmental dyslexia. In childhood the processes of learning to read, write, and spell are closely related. In essence they form a unity in which reading is the nuclear component, with retardation in the development of reading skills usually entailing a corresponding retardation in learning to write and spell. Consequently, children with developmental dyslexia only rarely show the dissociation between reading and writing or between reading and oral spelling which is so often seen in adult patients with acquired specific dyslexia. Another obvious difference between the two conditions is that the focal neuropathology of the dominant hemisphere which underlies acquired dyslexia is not demonstrable in developmental dyslexia.

However, there are also certain similarities which emerge when the two conditions are compared. First and foremost, the overt clinical picture is essentially the same in the two conditions; one finds in both a severe disability in visual language skills with no, or only very mild, impairment in auditory language skills. Secondly, as the contributions in this conference will show, clinical investigators have looked for and found a variety of behavioral deficits associated with developmental dyslexia just as their colleagues in the neurological clinic have with respect to acquired dyslexia. These deficits include impaired visual perception, insecure directional sense, poor development of "body schema" functions and defective auditory memory. Finally, none of the deficits which have been found to be associated with developmental dyslexia seems to offer by itself a satisfactory explanation for the disability just as none of them provides an adequate explanation for acquired specific dyslexia. Thus, we face the same problems of interpretation with respect to these two rather similar clinical conditions. It is reasonable to hope that progress in understanding one of them will advance our understanding of the other.

Developmental Dyslexia in Relation to Form Perception

Certainly the type of deficit which is mentioned most frequently as being associated with both acquired and developmental dyslexia is impairment in visual perception. This deficit is assumed, of course, to be general in nature, i.e., to apply to the perception of nonlinguistic and nonsymbolic visual stimuli as well as to symbolic material. By definition, gross visual object-agnosia is not present in acquired specific dyslexia. However, minor degrees of what is called "geometric form agnosia" (i.e., defective form discrimination) have often been reported. This observation has led some clinicians to conclude that the dyslexia is merely an attenuated form of visual agnosia, i.e., a more or less direct consequence or expression of impairment in form discrimination. The same conception has been advanced to account for developmental dyslexia. It is this thesis which we propose to examine in some detail.

The early students of developmental dyslexia generally made no mention of associated defects in visual form perception or in directional sense in their children with reading disability. On the contrary, they often took pains to emphasize the absence of any general or nonlinguistic defects which might account for the failure to learn to read. For example, James Hinshelwood (1917), in a final summary of his twenty years of experience with the condition, included "purity of the symptoms" as a basic definitional characteristic and essential for its diagnosis. He conceded that disabilities such as poor intelligence or defective auditory memory might well lead to a retardation in learning to read, but he drew a sharp distinction between such conditions and "true cases of congenital word blindness" in which "not only are the general intelligence, powers of observation, and reasoning unaffected . . . but the auditory memory is intact, and in many cases exceptionally good."

The first worker to investigate the possibility of a significant association between reading disability and perceptual (as distinguished from basic sensory) defects seems to have been Augusta Bronner (1917). In her book on the psychology of special abilities and disabilities, she explained the reading disability of one fifteen-year-old boy in terms of faulty visual memory and "visualization," the evidential basis for this being the boy's failure on the Binet memory-for-designs test and his testimony that he was unable to "visualize" the figures. Another case, again of a fifteen-year-old boy, was interpreted as being the resultant of poor auditory discrimination and memory. The boy's visual perception and memory were adequate but he was unable to repeat five digits, memory for auditorially presented syllables was poor and his oral speech was defective. Still other cases showed neither visual nor auditory defects. These cases, which Bronner found "most difficult to account for on the basis of such tests as seem to have a relationship to the factors in reading," led her "to wonder whether in reading there is not involved some subtle synthetic process, which, at the present time, we have no means of studying, but of defects which, nevertheless, are of extreme significance."

There followed two research reports which were to be rather influential in guiding subsequent thinking about the role of higher-level visual capacities in developmental dyslexia. The first was Lucy Fildes' study in 1921 of visual discrimination and memory in readers and nonreaders. She found that nonreaders showed some degree of disability in visual form discrimination and memory, not on a gross level to be sure, but in the perception of minor differences between visually presented figures. They also experienced difficulty in discriminating identical figures on the basis of spatial orientation alone, e.g., mirror images of the same figure. Similar results were secured in the auditory area, these findings leading her to conclude that developmental dyslexia "is but one aspect of a more general, yet still in itself specific, defect in either the visual or auditory regions or in both. All the nonreaders examined showed a reduction in the normal power in dealing with forms visually presented—especially when these forms were very like each other, their defect being shown most definitely in their failure to remember such forms."

In sharp contrast to these results of Fildes, quite negative findings were reported the following year by Gates (1922) in his study of the correlates of reading ability in school children. He could find no evidence that poor readers differed from good readers in respect to the visual discrimination of nonlinguistic material and he denied that visual perception or memory could account for reading disability. Indeed, he denied the validity of the concept of "general visual perception," asserting that "there are abilities to perceive words, digits, geometric figures, etc.; each of which is relatively independent of other perceptual abilities." Adopting a pluralistic approach, he implicated poor educational methods, unfavorable home influences, emotional factors, and defects of vision as determinants of retardation in reading development.

Thus, the battle was joined, with Fildes representing one point of view and Gates the other; it continues to this day. Since this is so, it is perhaps worth while to take a closer look at these two pioneer studies which were so important in determining both general attitudes about the nature of developmental dyslexia and, more specifically, conceptions of the significance of higher-level visual abilities in the disorder.

The study of Fildes dealt with the performances of twenty-six children who were judged to be particularly poor readers. All but one had Stanford-Binet IQs below 89. The IQs of more than 80 per cent of the subjects were below 80; exactly half of the group had

IQs below 70. They were compared with some good readers who are said by Fildes also to be intellectually subnormal. However, details are not given and it is impossible to tell how closely the factor of general intelligence was controlled in these comparisons. In any case, Fildes reported that there was no relationship between reading ability and intelligence level. The children were examined individually. There were, however, varying numbers in each experiment. The results are presented in terms of either percentages of various types of response or error scores without much indication of the extent of individual variation. Although the trends of the findings seem fairly obvious it is difficult for the critical reader to analyze them.

The study by Gates was quite different in nature. A much larger number of children was involved but the tests of visual perception were of the paper-and-pencil group type. The intelligence of the group was above average and there was no child with an IQ below 80 in it. In contrast to Fildes' results, a significant positive correlation between reading ability and intelligence was found. Over eight hundred correlation coefficients detail the relationships among the findings in this group of children whose reading achievement varied from one extreme to the other. Thus, although the investigation purported to have special reference to reading disability, it was actually an examination of relationships over the whole range of reading achievement in school children.

Comparing the two studies, one sees that different types of children were investigated in each, the subjects of Fildes' study being intellectually subnormal, those in Gates' study being intellectually normal. Fildes made a direct comparison of contrasting groups of good and poor readers while Gates correlated performances on various tasks with reading achievement as a continuous variable. Fildes examined her subjects individually while Gates utilized group tests. Given these differences in the groups tested, the designs of the studies, and the tests employed, it is not surprising that these two pioneer investigations yielded different results.

The concept that a disturbed directional sense underlies developmental dyslexia was elaborated by Orton (1937) in a series of studies beginning in 1925. Orton started from the observation that there appeared to be a striking tendency for dyslexic children to show a reversal in right-left (and, sometimes, up-down) orientation in reading letters or words, e.g., *b* for *d* or *saw* for *was,* and vice versa. So impressed was he with the importance of this phenomenon that he proposed the term *strephosymbolia* ("twisted symbols") as a designation for developmental dyslexia. He called the misreading of letters (typically reading a letter as its mirror-image) a "static" reversal. Since the misreading of words involves an inversion in the sequence or spatiotemporal ordering of letters, he designated this type of error as a "kinetic" reversal.

Orton evidently conceived of this impairment of directional sense as applying primarily to symbolic stimuli rather than to all visual stimuli. Thus, it was a perceptual deficit which was connected integrally with visual language function, not visual function in general. For example, one finds no mention in his 1937 monograph that directional sense is impaired when the dyslexic child is dealing with nonlanguage problems. Thus, he writes: "Functions other than reading but which incorporate a visual element are usually entirely normal. For example, visuomotor coordination may be excellent. . . . Visual recognition of objects, places, and of persons is quite normal, and interpretation of pictorial and diagrammatic material is frequently very good. Sense of direction is also often very well developed as in the case of one boy with such a marked reading difficulty that he could not understand any of the signboards along the way, who had nevertheless memorized routes so that he was the trusted guide for automobile trips."

Marion Monroe's classic monograph on reading disability (1932) appeared during this period when Orton was doing his work. Her final list of fifteen possible causative factors in reading disability includes both defective form perception and insecure directional sense. She assumed that the first type of disability ("lack of precision in discrimination of complex visual patterns") was reflected, in the child's reading, in the form of an inability to comprehend words as units although they might be recognized when they were spelled out. The second disability ("lack of precision in discrimination of spatial orientation") was assumed to reflect itself in the static and kinetic reversals described by Orton. However, Monroe merely postulated that these two perceptual deficits were significant correlates of developmental dyslexia. She employed no independent measures of form perception of directional sense as they applied to nonlinguistic material and did not adduce any empirical evidence that defective perceptual reactions of these types extended beyond the process of reading itself. In contrast, in dealing with such factors as motor speech defects and defective auditory word-discrimination, Monroe did show a significant association between these defects and developmental dyslexia.

There has been a good deal of empirical investigation of the question whether the dyslexic child does in fact show inferior visual form perception independent of his defective recognition of letters or words. The results have been inconsistent, but at least at times they have been suggestively positive. The findings of three recent studies which did yield positive results will be cited for purposes of illustration.

Galifret-Granjon (1952) reports that the performances of dyslexic children on the Bender Visual Motor Gestalt Test proved to be inferior to those of normal readers; the differences were observed to be more marked in the younger age groups (7 to 10 years) than in the older (11 to 13 years). On an incomplete figures test (Rey), the younger dyslexic children did less well than their controls but there were no differences among the older children in this respect. A slight inferiority in performance on the part of the younger dyslexic children was also observed in a "mixed figures" test (Poppelreuter). Essentially the same findings were secured on tests of constructional praxis, such as the Mannequin and Profile on the Arthur scale, the Goldstein-Scheerer "stick" test and the Kohs Block Designs. The dyslexics performed at a lower level than would be expected for their age; the differences were, however, more impressive at the younger age levels. It must be remarked that the dyslexic subjects in this study formed a very heterogeneous group which included mentally defective and obviously brain-damaged children as well as more or less "pure" cases with adequate intelligence. Moreover, direct comparisons with the performances of a control group were not always done, reference being made to published norms in some of the tests.

Although it does not actually deal with the clinical problem of reading disability, a recent study by Goins (1958) of the relationship between various visuoperceptive skills and reading achievement in first-grade children deserves mention because its results are being cited as evidence that defective visual form perception and insecure directional orientation are significant determinants of reading disability. In this study a variety of nonverbal tests of visual perception, including recognition of similarities and differences in pictures and abstract designs, completing designs from a model and recognition of incomplete pictures, were given to first-grade children relatively early in the school year and the findings correlated with the results of reading tests given both early and late in the school year. Most of the tests correlated positively and significantly with reading level, the coefficients ranging from .2 to .5. The correlation coefficient between over-all performance level on the fourteen tests of visual perception and reading level was .5. However, this fairly impressive finding loses at least some of its force when one considers that over-all performance level on the perception tests was also related to intelligence level (the correlation coefficient being about .3) and intelligence level was itself related to reading level (the correlation coefficient being about .35). Thus, when the factor of intelligence level is controlled, the "pure" relationship between visuoperceptive skill and reading ability in these first-grade children is still positive and significant but somewhat less close than the uncorrected correlation coefficient would suggest. Goins also explored the effects of special tachistoscopic training in visual perception on reading level, a procedure which is of particular interest to us because of its possible implications for treatment. This training had no significant influence on reading performance.

Still more recently, Lachmann (1960) has compared the performances of groups of normal children, dyslexic children, and emotionally disturbed children who were not dyslexic on the Bender Visual Motor Gestalt Test. Dividing the groups into younger and older subgroups, he found that the younger dyslexics (8 to 10 years old) performed more poorly than either the normal or emotionally disturbed children. However, this difference was not observable in the older subgroups (11 to 12 years old), all three subgroups performing at about the same level.

Balancing these positive results, there has been no dearth of studies which have yielded negative findings in respect to this question of a relationship between defects in visual form perception and developmental dyslexia. One might cite first the early study of Bachmann (1927), following closely upon that of Fildes, which investigated form perception under both conventional and tachistoscopic exposure conditions. No inferiority on the part of the dyslexic children was found. Similarly, Ombredane's (1937) intensive study of three older dyslexic children (12 to 14 years old) of adequate intelligence yielded negative results. Visual form discrimination and perceptual speed were found to be quite normal. More recently, Malmquist (1958), in a study of the relations between visuoperceptive abilities and reading skills in first-grade children, secured results which provide little support for the conclusions of Goins. The level of discrimination of abstract designs and pictures related positively to reading ability, but the correlations were very low (uncorrected coefficients = .11 to .25).

When one reviews these findings, one is impressed with the fact that, when differences in form perception between normal and dyslexic children are reported, they are observed to occur for the most part in younger children. In older children these differences either are not apparent or are present to only a small degree. Moreover, a good many studies (this is as true of those yielding negative results as of those with positive findings) have not exercised a sufficiently precise control of the factor of general intelligence to provide valid information about the specific or "pure" relationship between higher-level visual form perception and reading ability. Since these higher-level perceptual skills are correlated with intelligence (indeed they often enter into its very definition), an at least broad matching of groups on this global variable is a necessity.

My conclusion is that deficiency in visual form perception is *not* an important correlate of developmental dyslexia. By this I mean that, while it may be a determinant of the language disability in some cases, it is not a significant factor in the majority of cases. A certain level of visual discriminative capacity is obviously a necessary precondition for learning to read, and there is variation in the rate of development of these visuoperceptive skills in the early years of life. Significant retardation in development which extends into the early school years will then necessarily entail a corresponding retardation in learning to read; hence a relationship between the two sets of skills in younger school children will be discernible. But as the retardation in level of visual perception is overcome by the child, his reading level should improve correspondingly, at least under favorable circumstances. Thus, I should guess (and it is only a guess) that *transient* reading disability is often conditioned by a retardation in the development of higher-level visuoperceptive skills. (Longitudinal studies of children who show specific reading disability in the early grades of school should advance our understanding of this issue.) If visuoperceptive skills remain defective, then reading will also probably remain defective. But this factor accounts, I think, for only a very small proportion of cases of developmental dyslexia in older school children (i.e., above the age of ten). There remains the "hard core," consisting of dyslexic children whose difficulties are not ascribable to nonsymbolic visuoperceptive deficit.

Developmental Dyslexia in Relation to Directional Sense

As we have seen, Orton postulated that insecure directional orientation in the visual perception of symbols accounted in large part for developmental dyslexia. Although he himself apparently restricted the deficit to the child's transactions with language, the concept of directional confusion was soon extended to include the perception of nonsymbolic stimuli—a very natural development, since there seems to be no reason why directional confusion (usually in the form of right-left disorientation) should not apply also to any type of stimulus-situation which permits "mirror-image" responses. In recent years, the concept that directional confusion is the basis for developmental dyslexia has perhaps been stated most explicitly by the Danish neurologist, Hermann (1959), who describes the fundamental disturbance as being "a defect involving the categorical sphere of function which may be termed directional function. The directional disturbance is related to a failure of lateral orientation with reference to the body-schema, such that concepts of direction are either uncertain or abolished; the individual consequently has difficulty in orientating himself in extrapersonal space. This difficulty in orientation has particular consequences for the ability to operate with symbols such as letters, numbers and notes."

Investigation of the role of directional sense as a factor in dyslexia has proceeded along two lines. First, the ability to discriminate between different orientations of identical figures, and tendencies to reverse the conventional left-to-right orientation as well as temporal orientation in sequential stimulation have been assessed. Secondly, since directional sense has been related to the development of the body schema, the right-left orientation of normal and dyslexic children, with respect both to their own bodies and to those of other persons, has been examined.

The assessment of directional orientation in visual perception has often been included in the studies of form discrimination which we have already reviewed. It will be recalled that Fildes reported poor discrimination between identical forms in different orientations as well as defective form perception in her dyslexic subjects. Similarly, the test battery of Goins included a task which required the discrimination between the mirror-image forms of identical figures. Performance on this test correlated as closely with reading achievement in her first-grade children as did score on the total battery of fourteen tests. It also was as closely related to intelligence level as was score on the total battery. A recent study by Shepherd (1956) dealing with this question might also be mentioned. He reports that children with relatively poor oral reading skills showed a right-to-left orientation in free-hand drawing (e.g., drawing an arrow with its tip toward the left or a bird with its head toward the left) more frequently than did good oral readers. This right-to-left orientation tendency did *not* appear when the children copied abstract designs from a model.

Nevertheless, the story is very much the same as it is in the case of visual form perception. Other investigators have failed to adduce evidence to support the hypothesis of an unduly high incidence of insecurity or confusion in directional sense in dyslexic subjects. The ingenious procedures employed by Ombredane to test the hypothesis are perhaps worth mentioning. He had his dyslexic subjects copy graphic symbols without phonetic significance, a screen having been placed between the writing hand and the eyes so that the writing could not be guided by vision; the figures were reproduced in their normal orientation. Nor were reversed responses made when the subjects "read" Morse code aloud by sounding the visually presented dots and dashes in terms of short and long notes on a flute.

It is well known that the directional orientation of figures is often a matter of indifference to the preschool child. In each situation he must learn the conventional discriminations between the "right-side-up" and "upside-down" or "correct" and "mirror-image" orientations of stimulus-patterns. That this learning takes place over a number of years as the child encounters new and unfamiliar types of stimuli is evidenced by the frequency of reversal errors in the reading of first-grade children. Under pressure, the average first-grade child establishes these discriminations fairly readily. If, then, for one reason or another, these directional habits are not firmly established, the child's reading will suffer, for fluent reading requires a consistent left-to-right motor and perceptual orientation. On this basis, a negative relationship between insecure or inverted directional habits in visual perception and fluency in reading may well be expected; and it is reasonable to interpret this relationship to mean that poor directional sense plays a significant role in many cases of reading retardation.

However, this does not answer the question of the importance of the factor of directional sense in the severe and persistent disability which we designate as developmental dyslexia. Without necessarily denying the conception that reading ability is a continuous variable, we must nevertheless recognize that the backward reader may be quite different from the virtual nonreader, just as we recognize that the high-grade mental defective of IQ 75 and the low-grade defective of IQ 25 present quite different problems, although both are placed in the broad category of mental deficiency. In this connection, it is of interest that in Shepherd's study the important relationships which were found were between *oral* reading and directional reversal in drawing. On the other hand, performance on a silent reading comprehension test was not significantly related to the directional tendencies in drawing. In short, the disturbed directional sense seemed to be more closely associated with nonfluency in reading than with failure to appreciate the symbolic significance of written language.

The evidence that disturbed directional sense is a significant determinant of developmental dyslexia, as distinguished from mere relative backwardness in reading, is very sparse indeed. Whether continued investigation will strengthen the hypothesis is an open question. I am personally inclined to doubt that it will. For it seems to me that, in order for a directional disability to operate as the sole and sufficient cause of developmental dyslexia, it would have to be quite severe and to extend into diverse areas of behavior. The affected individual would be not only dyslexic but also would be expected to show spatial disorientation and praxic difficulties. A few dyslexics present this picture, but most of them do not.

Interest in the right-left orientation of dyslexics as applied to their own bodies or those of other persons is derived from the assumption that maturation of this aspect of the body schema is a prerequisite both for accurate right-left orientation of objects in space and for establishment of the consistent directional habits required for fluent reading. In assessing the significance of this factor in dyslexia, it is important to realize that "right-left orientation" is a hierarchical complex of abilities and that it is necessary to specify exactly what one means when one speaks of impairment in this area (Benton, 1959). For example, the average seven-year-old child is capable of correctly discriminating single parts of his own body in terms of right and left and to this degree can be said to possess "right-left orientation." At the same time, however, he will quite often fail to reverse his orientation in identifying single body parts on the confronting examiner and he may perform double-crossed commands (for example, "Put your right hand on your left eye") incorrectly. It is only somewhat later that he gains full appreciation of the right-left concept. This learning extends over several years before complete mastery is achieved. A ten-year-old child may correctly identify lateral body parts on the confronting examiner, showing thereby that he "knows" that a 180 degree reversal in orientation is required to make these discriminations. At the same time, his inability to handle both the "own body" and "other person" orientation systems simultaneously will be shown in his confusion on tasks that require him to place one of his hands on a designated body part of the examiner (e.g., his *right* hand on the examiner's *left* shoulder).

Intelligence level is significantly associated with all these levels of right-left orientation and particularly with the more complex performances. Hence, in studying right-left orientation in any clinical group, it is essential that account be taken of the factor of intelligence so that one may guard against the error of attributing distinctive performance characteristics to the diagnostic category when they can be explained quite adequately in terms of the more general factor.

Studies of children who are dyslexic (or at least are backward readers) suggest that an excessively high proportion of them do show defective right-left orientation on one or another level, (Harris [1957]; Hermann and Norrie [1958]; Benton and Kemble [1960]; Silver and Hagin [1960]). However, estimates of the actual incidence of defective orientation have varied widely—from a startling 92 per cent to an almost normal 6 per cent. When dyslexic and control children are matched for intelligence rating, a higher-than-average incidence of defective orientation is still found in the dyslexics, but the intergroup difference is not very marked. For example, in my own study, I found that six out of twenty dyslexic children (i.e., 30 per cent) showed deviant right-left orientation, as compared with two (i.e., 10 per cent) of the controls. Four of the six dyslexic children did not show a sheer *lack* of right-left discriminative ability but rather a *systematic reversal tendency*. That is to say, these children consistently discriminated their right and left body parts, even in the execution of double-crossed commands, but at the same time attached the wrong verbal labels to the parts. For example, when requested to place their right hand on their left eye, they would place their left hand on their right eye, etc. In an earlier study (Benton [1958]), I had found that this systematic reversal tendency was associated with a retardation in the development of language skills. Furthermore, children who showed systematic reversal in response more often failed to correct their orientation when identifying lateral body parts of the confronting examiner than did children whose discrimination followed the conventional lines. It seemed from these studies that dyslexia and backwardness in reading may be associated particularly with defect in the higher-level right-left orientation performances, i.e., those involving a conceptual or verbal element.

In the study of Harris, 38 per cent of the seven-year-old children with reading disability showed inferior right-left orientation, as compared with a base rate of 5 per cent in control children. However, the incidence of poor performance fell to 10 per cent in the eight-year-old reading cases and to 6 per cent in the nine-year-old cases. These findings suggest that the ability to discriminate right and left body parts plays a role in the early stages of learning to read and that lack of differentiation of this aspect of the body schema is associated with retardation in learning to read. However, this is not tantamount to saying that disturbances of the body schema play an important role in developmental dyslexia. This question remains open. It is true that Hermann and Norrie found a quite high incidence of defective right-left orientation in their dyslexic children and adults; but there is no indication that the decisively important factor of intelligence was controlled in their study. Silver and Hagin report that 92 per cent of their children showed defective right-left discrimination (as compared with zero incidence in the control group!); but their children were also behavior problems and showed disturbances in praxis as well as a variety of visuoperceptive and visuomotor difficulties and one cannot help but wonder whether the backward reading in their cases was simply a part-expression of a gross behavioral disturbance. In contrast, both Harris and I have found the incidence of right-left disorientation to be only slightly higher in dyslexics than in normal readers.

Concluding Remarks

We have seen that the literature on the role of form perception and directional sense in dyslexia is quite inconsistent in its indications. However, a good many of these inconsistencies can be resolved if account is taken of the factors of age and intelligence in interpreting the findings. A seven-year-old child who has not profited from a year of instruction in reading is called "dyslexic." So also is a ten-year-old child who is still reading at a first-grade level after three or four years of instruction. If, however, one declines to make the assumption that these children necessarily belong in the same category and one considers the younger and older children separately, the picture is clarified to a considerable degree. Inferior form perception, visuomotor skill and directional sense is associated with reading retardation in younger school children. However, as the investigations of Galifret-Granjon, Lachmann and Harris have shown, this association either disappears or is greatly attentuated when older dyslexic children are studied. A tenable (but not necessarily correct) conclusion is that the importance of these factors as specific determinants of severe and persistent dyslexia in children of adequate intelligence has been rather exaggerated. They may play a significant role in the early school years when the child is learning the rudiments of reading and hence are of major interest to the teacher and the school psychologist. In any case, they must always be included in the evaluation of a dyslexic problem. But it does not seem that they can be made to account for more than a small proportion of the cases of severe dyslexia presented by older school children. And this small proportion of cases will typically show such a variety of impairments in perception, praxis, and oral language that one wonders how "specific" their dyslexia is. This raises definitional questions which require discussion but which are beyond the scope of this paper.

With respect to indicated investigative work, it would seem that careful longitudinal studies extending over five or ten years should prove to be fruitful in testing the hypothesis I have put forth, namely, that these perceptual and directional factors are more important in the early learning of reading than in the persistent dyslexia which is of prime interest to the clinician. Beyond this, the finding that some dyslexics perform defectively on higher-level right-left orientation tasks which would appear to involve the operation of conceptual systems suggests that this type of performance should be further explored. It may be that such studies would show that the older dyslexic does show disturbed "form perception" and "directional sense" when the task requires implicit verbal mediation for optimal performance.

7

Dyslexia in Relation to
Cerebral Dominance

O. L. ZANGWILL

Introduction

Origin of the Concept. The notion of *cerebral dominance*—never, it may be said, a very precise one—owes its origin to the discovery that loss of speech (aphasia) almost always results from a lesion of the left hemisphere. Inevitably, this suggested a possible link with *handedness,* and the idea soon gained currency that both right-handedness and the lateralization of speech are due to an innate functional pre-eminence of the left hemisphere (Bouillaud [1864/5]; Broca [1865]). In left-handers, it was thought, the position is reversed, aphasia being therefore liable to result from a right-sided lesion. This was in fact demonstrated by Hughlings Jackson (1868, 1880), who appears to have been the first to describe aphasia in association with left hemiplegia in left-handed patients. At the same time, he was careful to point out that in not every case of aphasia associated with left hemiplegia seen by him had the patient been indisputably left-handed (Jackson [1868]). Further, cases began to multiply in which aphasia in left-handed patients appeared to be associated with lesions not of the right but of the *left* hemisphere. These were termed "crossed aphasia" (Bramwell [1899]). Such cases were, however, for many years regarded as exceptional and as not seriously challenging the validity of Broca's rule. Thus the *dominant hemisphere* came to be accepted as that which, with few exceptions, is contralateral to the preferred hand. This hemisphere has been supposed to "take the lead" in manual skill and in the control of articulate speech (Jackson [1869]).

Scope of Dominance. As the definition of new cerebral syndromes proceeded, the concept of cerebral dominance gradually became extended to cover other aspects of language. In particular, the work of Wernicke (1874) strongly suggested that speech in its receptive aspects could be lateralized to the left temporal lobe. Evidence was adduced that reading and writing evolve under control of the dominant hemisphere and may be selectively impaired by unilateral lesions (Broadbent [1872]; Bastian [1898]). Nor was the idea limited to language. In 1908, Liepmann attempted to relate certain higher disorders of movement (apraxia) specifically to lesions of the left hemisphere. In his view, this hemisphere may be said to "take the lead" in manipulative activities no less than in articulate speech. More recently, the idea of dominance has attracted fresh interest in connection with the differences in symptomatology associated with lesions of the two parietal lobes (Critchley [1953]). For instance, the syndrome of finger agnosia (Gerstmann [1924]) is almost always associated with lesions of the dominant hemisphere whereas visuospatial disorders appear more pronounced in cases in which the nondominant hemisphere is affected (Zangwill [1961]). There are also suggestions that equivalent lesions of the temporal lobes do not have equivalent effects (Bingley [1958]; Milner [1958]). Although it is always perilous to argue from "symptom" to "function," these differences in cerebral symptomatology are sufficiently striking as to suggest an important difference in the functional organization of the two hemispheres.

Two Meanings of Dominance. The idea of cerebral dominance has two aspects which have not always been kept distinct. In the first place, it implies the hypothesis that the central mechanisms subserving speech—and perhaps other higher functions as well—are located, predominantly at least, in one hemisphere. Put another way, it might be said that function is asymmetrically represented in the two halves of the brain so that equivalent unilateral lesions do not produce equivalent effects (Brain [1945]; Zangwill [1961]). In the second place, the idea of dominance has conveyed to some the notion that one hemisphere *exercises direct control* over its fellow in coordinated action. This particular interpretation of dominance seems to have arisen with Liepmann (1908), who inferred from his studies on apraxia that the right sensorimotor cortex is subject to control by the left in the execution of skilled actions. It reappears in the work of Travis (1931) who postulated a similar relationship between the motor speech zones in the two hemispheres. Unfortunately, no direct evidence of such a dominance relationship between the two hemispheres has been forthcoming, and studies of the effects of callosal section in man (Akelaitis [1943]; Smith [1945]) have rendered any simple conception of this kind exceedingly difficult to sustain.

Establishment of Dominance. It was predicted by Broca (1865) that extensive damage to the left hemisphere at birth would not preclude the acquisition of speech, thereby suggesting that the preeminence of this hemisphere is not wholly a matter of heredity. There can be no doubt that his prediction has been sustained. Extensive damage to the left hemisphere at birth or in early infancy does not prevent the development of speech (though it may of course delay it) and operative removal of the affected hemisphere at a later age is seldom followed by aphasia (Carmichael [1954]). Evidently, then, the right hemisphere has a potential capacity to subserve speech. Unfortunately, we know very little about the limits of this capacity beyond the fact that it appears to diminish rapidly with age and to be virtually lost with the advent of maturity.

It would appear, then, that what we call cerebral dominance reflects the development of asymmetrical functions in the two hemispheres. This process is to be envisaged as primarily one of maturation, though it is no doubt modified and reinforced by learning. There is evidence of a marked degree of equipotentiality of the two hemispheres at birth but a strong suggestion that this is rapidly lost with the acquisition of speech. No clear evidence has been adduced that one hemisphere exercises direct control over its fellow in speech or motor activity.

Handedness and Cerebral Dominance

Speech and Handedness. In the dextral adult, the traditional association between aphasia and lesions of the left hemisphere has not been seriously challenged. Indeed, in cases of brain injury sustained after the age of two, the incidence of aphasia in right-handed persons with lesions involving the right hemisphere only is so low as to be almost negligible. Penfield and Roberts (1959) report aphasia in only one of their 196 right-handed patients after operations on the right hemisphere; and Espir and Russell (1961) find only three such cases in a group of 221 right-handed patients with well-lateralized penetrating wounds of the right hemisphere. In the literature, it is true, there are a few striking cases of severe and persistent aphasia in dextrals with right-sided lesions (Ettlinger, Jackson, and Zangwill [1955]); but in a good many of these there is evidence of sinistral antecedents. For practical purposes, the probability of right cerebral dominance in a fully right-handed individual is so low that it may be disregarded.

In the case of the sinistral adult, and in those with various "mixed" patterns of laterality, the position is entirely different. As has been said, "crossed aphasia" in sinistrals was noted early (Paget [1887]; Bramwell [1899]), but was dismissed as exceptional. It is now clear, however, that aphasia in sinistrals may be expected to result more frequently from left-sided than from right-sided brain lesions (Humphrey and Zangwill [1952]; Goodglass and Quadfasel [1954]; Penfield and Roberts [1959]; Zangwill [1960]; Espir and Russell [1961]). I have reviewed the evidence elsewhere (Zangwill [1960]), and the facts are hardly open to doubt. The question is: What do they mean for the theory of cerebral dominance?

Are "Handedness" and "Brainedness" Independent? One answer to this question is that "handedness" and "brainedness" (i.e., the hemisphere in which speech is located) are essentially unrelated; that is to say, their incidence is independent. Several authors have suggested that this may be so. For example, Goodglass and Quadfasel (1954) write that "the tendency for language to center predominantly in the left hemisphere is in large measure independent of handedness." Penfield and Roberts (1959) make the rather cryptic statement that "brain function and handedness may be unrelated except by disease," suggesting that there is no true relation between dexterity and speech. Yet I do not believe that this necessarily follows from the evidence. As Bingley (1958) points out, if "handedness" and "brainedness" are wholly unrelated, we should expect to find a much higher proportion of "crossed aphasias" (i.e.; aphasias from lesions ipsilateral to the preferred hand) in dextrals than in fact we do. (The incidence of "crossed aphasia" in dextrals is unlikely to exceed one per cent). Similarly, we should on this hypothesis expect aphasia from right-sided lesions in left-handed patients to be excessively rare, whereas in fact it is relatively common. (The incidence of "uncrossed aphasia" in sinistrals appears to be about 30 per cent.) Indeed Bingley arrives at a correlation of .59 between "handedness" and "brainedness" which is certainly significant.

The Hypothesis of Bilateral Speech Representation. A second hypothesis is that speech in sinistrals is represented in *both* hemispheres, aphasia being liable to result from a lesion of either side (Conrad [1949]; Goodglass and Quadfasel [1954]; Hécaen and Piercy [1956]; Zangwill [1960]). This does not necessarily imply that sinistrals lack a dominant hemisphere, merely that unilateral representation of speech is typically less complete than in the dextral. In support of this view one may adduce the frequency of aphasia in sinistrals with lesions of either hemisphere, the frequency of mild or transitory aphasic syndromes in left-handed patients, and the finding that paroxysmal dysphasia in sinistrals is liable to occur with a focus in either hemisphere (Hécaen and Piercy [1956]). On the other hand, there is a good deal of evidence which goes strongly against the hypothesis. In the first place, Penfield and Roberts (1959) find no significant difference in the frequency of aphasia after operation on either the left or the right hemisphere as between left-handed and right-handed patients. In the second place, Espir and Russell (1961) report that the incidence of early aphasia after penetrating wounds of *either* hemisphere is no higher in sinistrals than in dextrals. And in the third place, experience with the Wada sodium amytal test indicates that in left-handed patients (or in those with uncertain handedness) transitory aphasia is produced in the great majority of cases by injection on one side only—as a rule the left though sometimes the right (Perria, Rosadini, and Rossi [1961]; Milner in a personal communication to the author). These findings effectively disprove the hypothesis that aphasia in sinistrals results indifferently from a lesion in either hemisphere.

At the same time, it cannot necessarily be concluded that the cerebral organization of speech is precisely the same in sinistrals as in dextrals. There is fairly convincing evidence that aphasia following injury of the left hemisphere disappears more rapidly and more completely in sinistrals (or in those with sinistral antecedents) than in fully right-handed patients (Luria [1947]; Subirana [1958]). This might suggest that in the sinistral the right hemisphere retains in adult life some, at least, of the capacity to subserve speech which it undoubtedly possesses in infancy. If so, it might be concluded that unilateral specialization is less complete in sinistrals than in dextrals and permits a higher degree of functional restitution after damage to the dominant hemisphere.

Implications for Dyslexia. The issues discussed above are of some significance in relation to the study of developmental language disorders. As is well known, Orton's attempt to explain these disorders in terms of faulty cerebral dominance made great play with the frequency of left-handed and ill-lateralized children in the dyslexic population (Orton [1934; 1937]). His hypothesis can be sustained only if we can accept that handedness is in fact related to language laterality and can be used as an index of hemisphere dominance. Although cerebral dominance in sinistrals presents some awkward problems, it seems reasonable to conclude that some intrinsic connection exists between handedness and the cerebral organization of speech.

Cerebral Dominance in Dyslexia

The Problem. It has been pointed out over and over again that many backward readers are left-handed, ill-lateralized, or exhibit inconsistence of preference as between hand, foot and eye (Monroe [1932]; Burt [1950]; Vernon [1957]). Yet opinion differs greatly as regards both the incidence and the significance of such anomalies and a few investigators have denied outright that there is any correlation between atypical laterality and backwardness in reading (Hallgren [1950]; Hermann [1959]). Others have stated that a correlation exists but is without special significance (Burt [1950]). At all events, it is obvious that not all backward readers are ill-lateralized and that many individuals with odd or inconsistent lateral preferences learn to read normally.

As I see it, the problem is not simply one of correlation. Backwardness in reading can be due to so large a number of possible causes (Vernon [1957]) that it obviously should not be regarded as a unitary condition. For this reason, I am skeptical of inquiries, the purpose of which is merely to compare the incidence of atypical laterality in matched groups of backward and normal readers (Hilman [1956]). It is surely more fruitful to ask whether forms of reading backwardness exist in which anomalies of laterality are especially prominent. If any such be found, it can then be asked whether there are any associated disabilities which might suggest delayed or incomplete maturation of cerebral function. In this way, one or more syndromes might be defined which might permit of explanation in terms of failure to establish normal cerebral dominance.

Incidence of Atypical Laterality in Dyslexia. Although an excess of left-handedness among children with developmental dyslexia has been noted by some authors (Orton [1937]; Bakwin [1950]; Zangwill [1960]), by far the most frequent finding is that of *weak, mixed or inconsistent lateral preferences* (Orton [1937]; Macmeeken [1939] Galifret-Granjon and Ajuriaguerra, [1951]; Harris, [1957]; Ingram, [1959; 1960]). For example, Ingram and Reid (1956) have called attention to a marked lack of consistent hand-preferences in 71 per cent of a group of patients diagnosed as cases of developmental aphasia, nearly all of whom gave evidence of severe disability in reading and writing. Harris (1957) reports a significantly higher proportion of instances of "mixed handedness" in a group of dyslexic children as compared with a randomly selected control group. Left-handedness has also been stated to occur in families with an appreciable proportion of dyslexics (Orton [1937]; Barger, Lavin, and Speight [1957]; Ingram [1959]; Zangwill [1960]). Taken together, these findings might suggest that delayed or incomplete lateral specialization of cerebral function is closely linked with backwardness in reading.

At the same time, there can be no doubt that a fair number of dyslexic patients are fully dextral and have no family history of sinistrality or ambidexterity (Ingram [1960]). It would therefore seem expedient to inquire whether dyslexia in ill-lateralized individuals differs in any significant way from dyslexia presenting in individuals who are fully lateralized. So far as I am aware, no such comparison has as yet been undertaken. In my own experience, I have been struck by the frequency of retarded speech development, defects of spatial perception, motor clumsiness, and related indications of defective maturation in cases of dyslexia presenting in ill-lateralized (and some left-handed) children (Zangwill [1960]). In dyslexia presenting in fully right-handed children (without familial sinistrality), on the other hand, I have been more impressed by the comparative "purity" of the disorder. It is in these latter cases, perhaps, that a specific genetical factor, as adduced by Hallgren (1950) and Hermann (1959), might plausibly be assumed.

Ambiguous Handedness in Young Children. A recent study by Naidoo (1961) on the language ability of healthy children selected for study solely on the basis of handedness may prove to have considerable relevance to the dyslexia problem. A group of 418 randomly selected children (239 boys and 179 girls) aged four years, nine months to five years, eleven months was given a battery of ten conventional handedness tests and then divided into three groups on the basis of the results. These groups were right-handed (360 children), left-handed (38 children), and ambiguously-handed (20 children). The children in the third group were matched with regard to age, sex, and type of school with twenty strongly right-handed and twenty strongly left-handed children drawn from each of the other two groups. These 60 children were then carefully studied with regard to birth history, familial sinistrality, rate of speech development and intelligence-test level. It was found that the children with ambiguous handedness were, as a group, significantly inferior to the other two groups in verbal intelligence-test level. They also tended to have a history of slow speech development and a higher incidence of complications at birth. The incidence of familial sinistrality in this group was, however, the same as in the left-handed group. Although it is too early to say whether these groups will also differ in scholastic performance, it would appear *prima facie* likely that the group of ambiguously-handed children will come to present an appreciable proportion of reading problems.

Cerebral Dominance in Dyslexia. On balance, the evidence suggests that an appreciable proportion of dyslexic children show poorly developed laterality and that in these there is commonly evidence of slow speech development. Other defects noted in many (though certainly not all) of the cases include poor drawing and copying, weakness in spatial orientation, and uncertain discrimination of right and left. If poorly developed laterality can be linked with incomplete cerebral dominance, it might be said that these patterns of disability reflect faulty establishment of asymmetrical (i.e., normally lateralized) functions in the two hemispheres. What we must do now is to consider whether this maldevelopment is constitutional, i.e., genetically determined, or whether it is due to exogenous factors, e.g., minimal brain injury at birth. We have also to consider why all ill-lateralized children do not exhibit backwardness in reading.

It is extremely difficult to understand why some ill-lateralized children have reading problems and others—almost certainly the great majority—do not. The first explanation that springs to mind is that both poorly developed laterality and reading backwardness where present together are due to the effects of an actual cerebral lesion. In cases with early damage to the left hemisphere, shift of hand-preference (either complete or partial) is not, of course, uncommon. Moreover, slow speech development and backwardness in reading are commonly found in such cases and may well be due to partial transfer of speech to the right hemisphere. This explanation is supported by evidence of focal left hemisphere EEG abnormality or minimal neurological lateralizing signs in a small proportion of dyslexic children (Ettlinger and Jackson [1955]). At the same time, it obviously accounts for but a very small minority of children with reading problems.

A second explanation is that a certain proportion of children with ill-defined laterality have in addition a constitutional weakness in maturation. This is perhaps suggested by the not infrequent incidence in dyslexia of nonspecific EEG abnormality (Statten [1953]) or minimal signs of diffuse neurological dysfunction (Rabinovitch, Drew, De Jong, Ingram, and Withey [1954]; Cohn [1961a]). Why this should occur in the absence of acquired brain damage is obscure, but it is possible that a genetical factor controlling handedness and cerebral dominance is involved.

A third explanation is that individuals lacking strong and consistent lateral preferences (and perhaps also those with sinistral antecedents) are particularly vulnerable to the effects of *stress* (Zangwill [1960]). For instance, minimal brain injury at birth may affect more severely those who show no strong tendency to lateral specialization. In this connection, it is noteworthy that Naidoo's (1961) group of children with anomalous handedness gave evidence of an excess both of familial sinistrality and of complications at birth. It is also noteworthy that a history of early brain illness or minor epilepsy is not uncommon among ill-lateralized dyslexic children (Zangwill [1960]). At the same time, no controlled study has yet been undertaken of the comparative incidence of stressful events (traumata) in the history of ill-lateralized children with and without reading disability. It would therefore be premature to conclude that the ill-lateralized child is of necessity more greatly handicapped in response to accidents of circumstance.

It is difficult to arrive at any very clear-cut conclusion. If, however, it is agreed that dyslexia presents more frequently among the ill-lateralized, and if lack of definite lateral specialization implies atypical cerebral dominance, it follows that atypical cerebral dominance is characteristic of a fair proportion of backward readers. The dyslexia itself may result from early brain injury, constitutional defect in maturation, or retardation secondary to stress. Indeed, it may well be due to a combination of these factors. At all events, fuller understanding of reading and its disorders must presuppose fuller understanding of the ways in which asymmetrical functions become established in the human brain.

8

The Anatomy of Acquired Disorders of Reading*

NORMAN GESCHWIND

To most educators and pediatricians, the term *dyslexia* means the failure to acquire the ability to read; it is this disturbance which is the focus of interest of this volume. It is worth recalling that historically the first reading problems to have been investigated were cases of the *loss* of the ability to comprehend written language, and it is therefore common practice among neurologists to distinguish *acquired* dyslexia or alexia from their *congenital* counterparts.

The distinction between these acquired disturbances and the congenital dyslexias is not an academic one. Remarkably restricted lesions in the left cerebral hemisphere of the adult may cause permanent severe disabilities. By contrast, total destruction of the

* The researches described here were supported in part by a grant (No. M-1802) to the Section of Psychology, Massachusetts Institute of Technology from the National Institute of Mental Health, United States Public Health Service.

In the ensuing discussion, a certain number of neuroanatomical terms will be used that may be unfamiliar to those without special training. Such readers are advised to begin by reading the Appendix to this paper, p. 129, where a brief outline of the necessary information is presented.

left·hemisphere in early childhood ordinarily does not prevent acquisition of language. It seems clear that the distribution of pathology in the congenital disturbances of language must involve something other than what is involved in the aphasias of adults.

Very uncommonly, the acquired disabilities are of functional psychiatric origin (hysterical *blindness* is much more common). In nearly all cases the disability results from damage to the brain readily distinguished at post-mortem examination and the study of such lesions has been the most important technique for studying the parts of the nervous system involved in the comprehension of visual language in adults. An acquaintance with them is indispensable to any investigation of the apparently more elusive mechanisms involved in the failure to learn to read.

Three situations stand out prominently in which patients may lose the ability to read.[1] The most common is Wernicke's aphasia, in which the patient shows a severe incomprehension of both spoken and written language, together with a characteristic speech pattern (fluent speech which is often totally incomprehensible as the result of use of many distorted or incorrect words and extensive circumlocutions), and an inability to write correctly. A more restricted and less common syndrome is that of "pure word blindness with agraphia." The most restricted syndrome and the one whose mechanism I will discuss at some length is that of "pure word blindness without agraphia."

Before discussing this syndrome, the first question, oddly enough, must be whether I have a topic for discussion. Distinguished authors have disputed the existence of this entity. On the opposite side one finds equally distinguished adherents—Dejerine (1892); Bastian (1898); Holmes (1950); Symonds (1953); Warrington and Zangwill (1957); Hécaen, Ajuriaguerra, and David (1952); Alajouanine, Lhermitte, and Ribaucourt-Ducarne (1960). Some time ago those of us in the Aphasia Unit of the Boston Veterans Ad-

---

[1] Throughout this presentation the word *read* is used in the narrow sense of "ability to comprehend language presented visually" and not at all in the sense of "ability to read aloud." Even in the neurological literature the two meanings are often confused. Many patients who cannot read aloud comprehend the written word correctly.

ministration Hospital decided to review carefully individual case reports of this condition in the attempt to decide for ourselves whether it was justifiable to isolate the condition of "pure word blindness without agraphia."

We did not have to look far. The first reported case with a post-mortem examination is that of Dejerine (1892). Inexplicably this is a neglected paper. It is not mentioned in several works on aphasia. Where cited, it is often misquoted or even dismissed. Its value can be stated briefly. The careful description of the clinical picture has been confirmed more than once and it established an anatomical localization which has also been repeatedly confirmed. It is, in fact, a masterpiece of neurological clinicopathological correlation.

Dejerine's patient was an extremely intelligent 68-year-old man who, on October 25, 1887, suddenly observed that he could no longer read a single word. He was examined first by Landolt (a distinguished ophthalmologist and a pioneer in physiological optics) and the original findings were confirmed by Dejerine repeatedly over the next four years.

The patient had a visual acuity of 8/10, spoke fluently without error, and understood all spoken speech. Objects were named perfectly, including pictures of technical instruments in a catalogue. He could identify his own morning newspaper by its form but could not read its name. On presentation he could not identify a single letter by name. The only written material he could read was his own name. Writing was correct, both spontaneously and to dictation, but what was written could not be read back. As Dejerine commented, his writing was rather like that of a blind man, larger than normal and with poor orientation of the lines.

Although the reading of isolated letters was impossible, the patient could identify them by name after tracing their contours with his finger; if the examiner formed letters by moving the patient's hand through the air, he could name the letters produced in this way. This phenomenon had been described earlier in similar patients and many patients since then have shown the same finding.

A rather surprising contrast was the fact that even at the beginning of the illness, he could recognize individual Arabic numerals, but had trouble in reading several numbers simultaneously and in doing arithmetic calculations. With the passage of time all his difficulties in reading Arabic numerals and in doing even the most complex written calculations disappeared while his difficulties in reading letters persisted unchanged. Roman numerals were not tested. (Later observers have frequently confirmed the superiority in reading Arabic numerals in these patients, while Roman numerals seem to show the same difficulties as other letters.)

Like the other examples of this syndrome, this case showed a right hemianopia. Another frequently observed finding is a difficulty in color vision in the retained left visual field, but this is not mentioned by Dejerine.

The remarkable discrepancy between the loss of letters and preservation of numbers arouses one's interest in other visual symbols. The patient who had been a skilled musician now showed a total inability to comprehend musical notation, but could write a scale or particular notes to command. The ability to sing and play instruments was unimpaired.

The patient was observed carefully over the next four years. During this time he continued actively and very successfully in business, kept on writing, played cards skillfully, and learned and performed new music by ear. He had no difficulty in orientation even when going to strange parts of Paris.

On January 5, 1892, another cerebral vascular accident left him with paraphasic speech and incapable of writing. He died at 10 A.M. on the sixteenth of January and an autopsy was performed in the patient's home by Dejerine, twenty-four hours after his death.

Dejerine gave a careful description of the external appearance of the cerebral hemispheres and of the internal appearances as revealed by gross horizontal sections. There was no report of the microscopic findings in the lesions in this original publication, but these appeared in a later paper and in his monumental work on the anatomy of the brain. They fully confirmed the impressions he had drawn from observation of the gross specimen and supported his theoretical conclusions.

Two major lesions were found in the brain (Figures 1-4). There was the recent lesion (with which the patient had become paraphasic and agraphic) involving the angular gyrus and adjacent portions of parietal lobe and temporoparietal junction. It showed the characteristic features of a recent lesion: there were signs of both white and red infarction, in the absence of atrophy of the involved gyri, ingrowth of new vessels, yellowish coloration, thickening or adherence of the meninges. The older lesion (which is the one that is of major interest here since it is the one causative of the clinical picture I have been discussing) had caused destruction of the medial and inferior aspects of the occipital lobe. This showed the characteristic appearance of a lesion of considerable age with narrowing and atrophy of the gyri. The white matter of the occipital lobe was yellow and shrunken. In addition, there was a region of old destruction of white matter in the splenium of the corpus callosum.

In discussing the significance of the pathology, let us confine ourselves to the older lesion whose effects were apparent to Dejerine. He pointed out that for a word to be seen as language and not merely as an arbitrary design, there must be a connection between the visual centers in the occipital cortex and the language areas in the left hemisphere. But, in this patient, the destruction of the left occipital cortex and the resultant right hemianopia made it necessary for the patient to see only in his left visual field and hence, with his right occipital cortex. In this situation, for reading, it is necessary to have connections going from the right occipital cortex across the corpus callosum and to the left-sided language areas in the posterior temporal region. Dejerine argued that the extensive destruction of white matter in the left occipital lobe in this case would destroy the connecting fibers from the right occipital cortex. He thought that this destruction alone would suffice to disconnect the right visual area from the language areas without having to bring in the lesion of the splenium of the corpus callosum. There is good reason, however, to believe that the lesion of the corpus callosum did contribute significantly to the disconnection postulated by Dejerine. The anatomical evidence supports strongly the view that fibers from the occipital lobes to the corpus callosum run in the splenium where they are rather tightly packed.

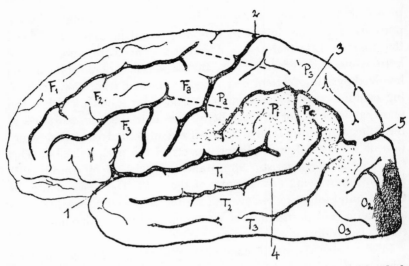

Figure 1.   Left hemisphere of Dejerine's patient, lateral view. The dark area in the occipital lobe represents the old region of destruction, the stippled area the recent lesion. 1 = Sylvian fissure; 2 = Rolandic fissure; F_3 = third frontal gyrus; T_1 = first temporal gyrus; Pc = angular gyrus. Reproduced from Dejerine (1892).

It is worth commenting here that Dejerine's anatomical conclusions from this case are frequently misquoted. A frequent statement is that he attributed this syndrome to a lesion of the angular gyrus. In fact, he carefully denied this. He had shown a year earlier that a lesion of the angular gyrus caused the syndrome of pure word blindness with agraphia and indeed, he thought that it was specifically disconnection of the right visual cortex from the left angular gyrus which led to pure word blindness without agraphia.

There is one feature of the clinical picture which is very compatible with the idea of a specialized disconnection. This is the fact that although letters could not be read by this patient when presented visually, they could be "read" when they were traced on his hand or when his hand was moved over the outline of a letter. This stimulation when presented to the right hand would go to the left sensory cortex and thence readily to the speech areas; when

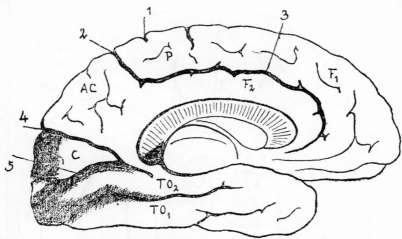

Figure 2. Left hemisphere, medial view. The structure marked by radiating lines is the corpus callosum, the posterior end of which (the splenium) is seen to contain an area of old destruction. 5 = calcarine fissure, along the lips of which lies the visual cortex, which is shown as involved in the area of old destruction. Reproduced from Dejerine (1892).

presented to the left hand, it would go across the corpus callosum (anteriorly to the splenium) from the right hemisphere and thus reach the speech areas. This preservation of tactile or kinesthetic "reading" in pure word blindness without agraphia contrasts to its loss in pure word blindness with agraphia. The latter syndrome is the result of a lesion of a cortical area which somehow functions in the operations done on visual language; once destroyed, it is obvious that comprehension of written language is lost regardless of its mode of presentation; but, by a suitably placed lesion one can specifically disconnect from this cortical area visually presented material alone, while preserving the transmission of somesthetically presented stimuli.

A few years later, Bastian (1898) reviewed two more cases (in addition to Dejerine's) which had come to post-mortem and had shown similar clinical and pathological findings and led him to defend essentially the same mechanism.

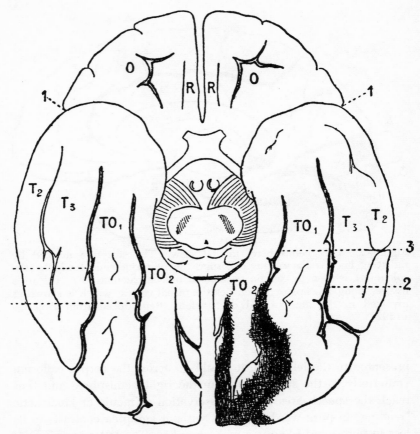

Figure 3. Cerebral hemispheres, seen from below. Reproduced from Dejerine (1892).

Foix and Hillemand (1925) advanced further evidence in support of a mechanism of disconnection and, in particular, of the importance of the lesion in the splenium. They had found that, in a case of destruction of the left occipital lobe with preservation of the splenium, there was no word blindness, despite the presence of the expected right hemianopia. By contrast, two cases which at post-mortem showed destruction of the splenium in addition to that of left visual cortex had manifested pure word blindness. The

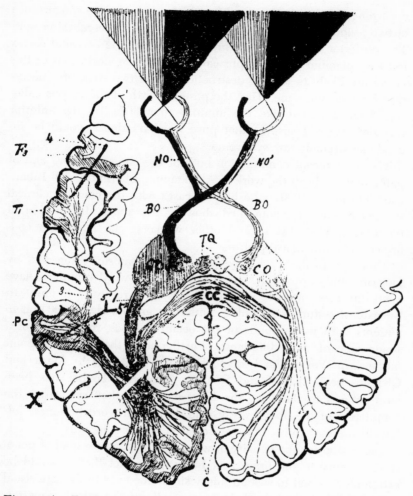

Figure 4. Diagrammatic horizontal cross section of cerebral hemispheres, illustrating the mechanism of pure word blindness without agraphia. NO = left optic nerve and NO′ = right optic nerve. C = left and right calcarine cortex, shown destroyed on the left (oblique lines); Pc = left angular gyrus (when destroyed as shown here alexia with agraphia results; this region is intact in pure alexia without agraphia); X = large lesion in white matter of left occipital lobe destroying fibers from the right visual cortex going to the left angular gyrus; cc = corpus callosum (although no lesion is shown here, a lesion here will be easily as effective as the lesion at X in disconnecting the right visual cortex from the left angular gyrus). Reproduced from Dejerine (1892).

occurrence of this syndrome, dependent as it is on the concurrence of two lesions, is a result of the arrangement of the cerebral vessels. The posterior cerebral artery supplies not only the occipital cortex but the splenium of the corpus callosum. Hence, occlusions of this vessel are likely to lead to destruction of the two structures necessary for this syndrome. Had the posterior fifth of the corpus callosum been supplied like the anterior four fifths by the anterior cerebral artery, I suspect that pure word blindness would be indeed an extremely rare syndrome.

The most recent confirmation both of the clinical picture and of pathology has been the work of Alajouanine, Lhermitte, and Ribaucourt-Ducarne (1960) who had six cases with the classical clinical syndrome, one of whom died showing the above distribution of pathology. They list several other workers who have also confirmed the pathological picture.

There is further evidence for the mechanism suggested by Dejerine and supported here. Cases of pure word blindness have been due most often to vascular disease and rarely to trauma. In the extensive studies of Teuber, Battersby, and Bender (1960) on 46 patients with war wounds of the occipital lobes, there was not a single case of word blindness. Furthermore, these authors point out that in World War I, no such cases were found by Marie and Chatelin or Wilbrand and Saenger. Professor Teuber has been kind enough to show me the notes on one patient seen after the completion of the above study who developed word blindness following trauma which, however, cleared in a few months.

The reason for the paucity of word blindness as a sequel of penetrating injury to the brain is, I believe, the fact that it would be extremely unusual to sustain injury simultaneously to the left visual cortex and the splenium of the corpus callosum. A missile penetrating the splenium would probably enter the upper brain stem and almost certainly lead to the patient's death.

The evidence from neurosurgical procedures lends further support to the argument. Hécaen, Ajuriaguerra, and David (1952) describe seven patients who underwent occipital lobe resection, all very extensive. Every one of these patients developed pure word-blindness, but in every case the disability cleared up within six months. (It is interesting, however, that all of these patients found reading unpleasant after their recovery.) If pure word blindness were the result of a lesion of some cortical region of the occipital lobe alone, permanent word blindness should have been seen in some of these cases. In contrast to the recovery of these patients is the fact that cases of this disorder that have a vascular origin have a very poor prognosis for recovery. The only difference between the vascular and surgical cases is the preservation of the splenium in the latter. Presumably the fibers from the right occipital lobe to the speech areas are so tightly packed in the splenium that they are more effectively destroyed here than they are by even a very extensive lesion of the white matter of the left occipital lobe.

The above suggested mechanism has further implications. If the splenium alone were destroyed, words presented in the *right* visual field should be read normally, but the patient should be word-blind for words presented in the *left* visual field. Two papers have presented such cases. Thus, Trescher and Ford (1937) found that a patient whose splenium had been sectioned for removal of a third ventricle tumor could not read letters in the left visual field although the standard visual field examinations were normal, nor could she name wooden letters placed into her left hand. On the other hand, objects placed in the left hand were named correctly and two-point discrimination was normal in this hand. Maspes (1948) presented two further cases in whom the splenium of the corpus callosum was cut for removal of colloid cysts of the third ventricle. Both these cases developed alexia in the left visual field alone.

For the past fifteen years attribution of clinical symptomatology to lesions of the corpus callosum has been unpopular because of the negative reports of physiologists on the effects of callosal section and particularly as a result of the studies of Akelaitis and his co-workers (1941; 1943; 1944) on interruption of the callosum in man. However, Sperry (1961) and his colleagues have recently conclusively shown that dividing the callosum leads to profound changes in animals, if they are examined properly. Sperry showed that if one hemisphere is trained, the learned material is transferred to the opposite hemisphere by way of the corpus callosum. After section of the callosum, new material presented to one hemisphere is not transferred to the opposite side. In man, the testing situation is simpler than in the animal since language skills remain confined to the left hemisphere in normals. Hence, immediately following callosal destruction, appropriate testing should reveal defects if the right hemisphere is tested with language tasks. The effect of posterior section is to cut off the right occipital lobe from the language areas. Sections further forward should have more profound effect on the limbs. Elsewhere we have described the effects of more anterior involvement of the corpus callosum (Geschwind and Kaplan, [1962]). I would like especially to express my debt to Dr. Sperry whose work alerted me to the possible importance of callosal disconnection in humans.

The most serious objection to the mechanism discussed here arises from the aforementioned work of Akelaitis and his co-workers. In particular, he described six patients in whom the splenium was cut; in none of them was there any subsequent alexia in the left visual field. These six cases stand in contradiction to the case of Trescher and Ford (1937) and the two cases of Maspes (1948). There is at present no obvious means of explaining the discrepancy, although some suggestions may be made. One possibility is that the sections performed on Akelaitis's cases were less complete than those done on the patients of the other authors, but since none of the patients has had a post-mortem examination, this cannot be verified. Maspes pointed out that in five of the six cases studied by Akelaitis, cerebral lesions had been present from early childhood. Language skills might not have been sharply localized in the left hemisphere in these cases and callosal section would therefore have shown little effect. All of Akelaitis's cases were epileptics, while none of the contrasting group were. Could epilepsy favor the opening up of alternative pathways? This is a rather hazardous speculation which can only be mentioned here. Clearly, further observations are needed.

In this final section, I would like to turn to some more remote implications of the interpretation of pure word blindness without agraphia that has been defended here. First are its implications for the general problem of interpretation of the aphasias. Neurologists have frequently assumed that "mixed" aphasias were the result of mixtures of "pure" lesions. But, even the patient with pure word blindness with agraphia does not have the lesion of pure word blindness without agraphia "mixed" with another lesion. Very pure lesions may result only from disconnection from the language areas and the possibility still remains that lesions directly in the speech areas can never produce a "pure" syndrome (in the sense of an aphasic disorder confined to a single modality). This view gains added support from the fact that many researches over the years have supported a similar mechanism for pure word deafness, i.e., a lesion of the left Heschl's gyrus, with destruction of callosal fibers from the right Heschl's gyrus, with no lesion in speech cortex. Hoff (1961) is the most recent investigator to have found pathological evidence for this mechanism.

The next point I would like to discuss is an apparent difficulty which arises from the mechanism for pure word blindness suggested above. Professor Davis Howes called my attention to the fact that none of the published cases of pure word blindness has had the symptom of so-called optic aphasia. By this term is meant the inability to *name* a seen object although the subject recognizes it (as proven, let us say, by his ability to select it afterwards from a group), with retained ability to name objects by feel, sound, smell, or taste. If indeed the right occipital lobe is disconnected from the language areas, how can the subject *name* seen objects? Let me sharpen this point by noting that in the patient mentioned earlier studied by Mrs. Kaplan and myself, who shows evidence of anterior callosal disconnection, one finds an inability to name *letters* placed in the left hand, i.e., a "tactile alexia" of the left hand. He also shows an inability to name *objects* placed in the left hand although he can identify them nonverbally, i.e., he has the analogue to "optic aphasia" which has been called "tactile aphasia." Why does "optic aphasia" not accompany pure word blindness? One possible explanation is the straightforward anatomical one, i.e., that different pathways are used in naming an object, or more likely, that the sight of an object is much richer in associations than that of a letter and that thus eventually more anterior parts of the right hemisphere are stimulated whence pathways are found across the corpus callosum. Adolf Meyer (1950) supported essentially this latter version of the anatomical explanation.

There is another approach to the problem of the preservation of object-naming. Dr. Davis Howes and I have recently had the opportunity to study a patient with pure word blindness without agraphia who presented the classical clinical syndrome. In his paper in this symposium, Dr. Howes describes the studies that we have conducted, and in particular, he discusses the comparative data on object- and word-naming respectively. One possibility which emerges from these data is that while object- and word-naming may use the same pathways, object-naming may survive partial damage more effectively. The data do not clearly decide between the anatomic and functional explanations and this remains an interesting area for further investigation.

In closing, we can turn to the question of the possible relevance of what has been presented here to the problem of "congenital dyslexia." I think one can say with some assurance that the lesion described here is not the cause of congenital dyslexia. Children with this disturbance do not have hemianopias. Furthermore, even if such a lesion did rarely occur in a child under the age of six, I doubt that it would impair his ability to learn to read, or if he were already reading, I believe that the disability would be transient. The reason for this is the tremendous ability of the youthful nervous system to find alternative means of compensating for damage to localized areas, a faculty much attenuated in the adult. However, I suspect that I could guess the type of explanation that Dejerine *might* have given for congenital dyslexia. He would have argued that the angular gyrus acts in some specific way to process visual language, and that *bilateral* maldevelopment of this region would be the minimum substrate for difficulty in learning to read. Is this the true explanation? I do not believe that an answer is available. I would only suggest that we keep in mind the lesson to be learned from Dejerine of the importance of interweaving our functional with our anatomical knowledge.

A p p e n d i x

This brief appendix is designed to aid the reader of this paper who lacks a technical background in neuroanatomy. The reader should refer to the illustrations given in the paper while reading this section.

The two halves of the brain (the *cerebral hemispheres*) are connected by a large bundle of nerve fibers called the *corpus callosum,* which can be seen on the inner surface of the divided brain. The posterior end of this structure is called the *splenium.* The cerebral hemispheres consist of an outer mantle of *gray matter* which is called the *cortex* which consists of *nerve cells* and a central core of *white matter* which consists of nerve fibers coming from or going to the cortex. The white matter carries to appropriate areas incoming sensations from the periphery, interconnects different parts of the cortex and carries impulses to muscles out of the cortex.

There are certain distinct specializations of the cortex. Visual impressions go to the posterior end of the cerebral hemisphere, the *occipital lobes,* with the right side of the visual field being represented in the left occipital cortex and the left side in the right occipital cortex. Language functions are carried out only on the left side of the brain in most people in the areas marked in Figure 1 as F_3 which is in the *frontal lobe,* in the area marked T_1 which is in the *temporal lobe,* and in the area marked P_c (the *angular gyrus*) which is at the junction of the temporal, parietal, and occipital lobes.

The word *hemianopia* refers to a loss of vision in one half of the visual field. The *left* half of each retina receives the image from the *right* half of the visual field, since the incoming image from the visual field is inverted by the lens of each eye. The left half of each retina is connected to the left occipital lobe of the brain. Thus, a right hemianopia (for each eye) signifies impaired perception in the right visual field and results from destruction of the visual cortex in the left occipital lobe and vice versa for a left hemianopia.

9

An Approach to the Quantitative
Analysis of Word Blindness*

DAVIS HOWES

Disease of the brain provides a vitally important source of information for our understanding of language function because in the strict sense no comparative study of linguistic phenomena is possible. Other psychological functions, even the highest and most complex, exist in homologous forms in other species, and our knowledge of their physiological bases is largely derived from experiments with lower animals. In the case of language we are completely cut off from this source. Many lower species, it is true, possess elaborate signaling systems that are sometimes called languages. But none of these resembles human language even in a rudimentary way. Nor, so far as we can tell, are those areas of the brain homologous to those associated with language in the human used for analogous functions in other species. Human language, in sum, presents one of the sharpest discontinuities in all of evolutionary development. This fact contributes added fascination to the study of language as a biological phenomenon, but it also

* The research reported here was supported by Grant No. M-1802 from the National Institute of Mental Health, United States Public Health Service.

131

eliminates one of our most valued experimental methods of investigation.

If we are to exploit to the fullest the implications of various pathological states of language, it is essential that we develop methods for the quantitative description and analysis of language deficits. Fertile as clinical methods have proved in the hands of masters, they cannot long continue unaided to yield rich fruit from the same soil. We need to supplement them with more powerful tools. For something as richly varied and rapidly fluctuating as human language, observations must sooner or later be put on a systematic quantitative basis. Otherwise we are incapable of holding in mind at one and the same time the many different facets of the language process that we can observe. Over the past five years Dr. Geschwind and I have been developing methods of this kind for the analysis of aphasic language (Geschwind [1961]; Howes [1962]). Recently we have begun to explore the possibilities of adapting similar procedures to cases of pure word blindness, and it is these beginnings that I wish to discuss here. My remarks will be confined to acquired dyslexias in adults; as the measurement of reading difficulty is their central theme, however, I hope they will also be of interest for the study of developmental dyslexias, which, though they may represent fundamentally different neurological disorders, present similar phenomena for measurement.

The paper is divided into four parts. In order to illustrate what I mean by quantitative analysis, which is not quite the same thing that is often meant by that term, I shall begin by briefly describing some of our research on aphasia. Aphasia is a phenomenon intimately related to word blindness, and it should not seem an unnatural point of departure for a consideration of word blindness. But the main reason for beginning my discussion with that topic is rather that our methods, and the reasoning that lies behind them, can better be illustrated by work that is well in progress than by our initial efforts on word blindness itself. The next section of the paper is devoted to the theoretical background for our use of analogous methods in the study of word blindness. The main technical obstacles are also taken up there. A third section presents the results of our initial experiments with word-blind patients and discusses some of their implications. In the final section I return to a theoretical problem concerning the mechanism for word blindness discussed by Dr. Geschwind in his paper in this symposium: namely, why is object perception preserved in these patients for whom word perception is almost completely absent?

I

Quantitative analysis is a term often used with reference to psychological tests of the usual sort, long familiar in neurological practice and research, where numbers are generated by counting the number of separate items the patient can pass in a test made up of many items. Such tests are extremely useful for many purposes, and I do not want to dwell on their shortcomings. But it is important to recognize that the numbers derived from them do not represent measurements of the trait or function being tested in the same sense that, for example, the numbers taken from a meter stick represent measurements of length. Strictly speaking, such tests do not represent a quantification of the trait or function at all.

What is meant by quantitative analysis here goes considerably beyond the psychological test of this type. It requires that we know some general empirical law governing the psychological function in which we are interested and that we be able to express that law, at least to first approximation, in the form of an equation containing only a small number of free parameters.

Consider the question of vocabulary size in aphasia. On listening to the typical patient with Broca's aphasia, it seems immediately obvious that the patient's vocabulary has been diminished. Yet the patient's rate of speaking is also slowed, and it is quite possible that our judgment of a diminished vocabulary may only reflect the fact that we hear fewer words from him in a given period of time. Appearances are often deceiving in such matters. To decide the question we must appeal to measurement.

One can, of course, attack the question by constructing tests of verbal capacity of the usual kind. One might, for example, present him with a list of test words for recognition or definition, as is often done in vocabulary studies of school children. But the results of such tests depend on the particular selection of words, the areas of the patient's vocabulary strength, and the criterion of recognition or definition, among other factors. They can, therefore, give a very misleading indication of the relative size of the patient's vocabulary. Furthermore, the scores obtained from such tests are arbitrary numbers, and there is no theoretical basis by which a meaningful measure of vocabulary size can be derived from them. Then, too, if a patient has difficulty understanding instructions, he may not be able to perform at all on the test, though he may use an extensive vocabulary in other situations. In cases of aphasia, therefore, estimates of vocabulary size based on data from verbal tests of this kind are extremely difficult to interpret.

For a more satisfactory measure of vocabulary, we may make use of an empirical law established by G. K. Zipf some twenty-five years ago. In its most general form, Zipf's law states that the distribution of word frequencies calculated from any *ad libitum* sample of language always has the same mathematical form. That is, the curve describing the proportion of the sample composed of words occurring 1, 2, 3, . . . times in that sample always conforms to a single equation. Zipf himself suggested a type of equation that is not very satisfactory either on empirical or theoretical grounds, but his work clearly established the existence of a regularity. Figure 1 presents illustrative data from a very large sample (4.5 million words) fitted to a better equation, the logarithmic normal.

The data from many different languages representing distinct language families from all over the world have been found to conform to this equation. Written as well as spoken language from all normal subjects that have been tested yield this form of word-frequency distribution without exception. The form of the equation does not depend on the subject matter or the situation. Note that the equation depends on the number of words occurring with every possible frequency. Hence, it is not greatly affected by circumstances that increase the number of words occurring just once, such as lists of objects or names, for these affect only a single point on the curve.

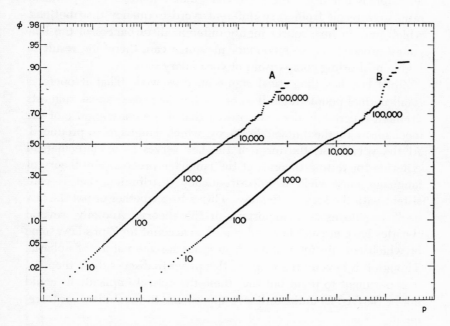

Figure 1. Word-frequency distributions for two large samples plotted on logarithmic-normal coordinates. Abscissa (p): word frequency plotted on a logarithmic scale. Ordinate (ϕ): proportion of sample composed of words of frequency p or less plotted on a normal probability (probit) scale. A: Lorge Magazine Count (English, 4.5 million words). B: Kaeding Count (German, 11 million words). Curve B has been shifted two logarithmic units to the right to avoid overlap.

From the word-frequency distribution we can, if we wish, derive the cruder vocabulary measures like the number of different words in a sample of stated size (type-token ratio), or the various redundancy numbers based on information theory. The converse, however, is not true: the same redundancy number or type-token ratio may result from very different word-frequency distributions, which may in turn reflect highly different disturbances of the language process. These secondary measures can, therefore, result in highly misleading comparisons of vocabulary size.

Zipf's law has theoretical significance as well. That it operates in all normal people regardless of the language they speak suggests (though it certainly does not prove) that it is a consequence of the mechanism in the human brain by which language is produced. At the very least, the form of the law serves as a mathematical criterion for testing theories of the language process: any theory of language must yield a word-frequency distribution that is consistent with the form of the law. This is true whether or not the law itself be intrinsically important in the theory. Actually, several theories have already been advanced to account for Zipf's law, some of which contain interesting suggestions for the nature of aphasia. Though it is beyond the scope of this paper to discuss these theories, it is pertinent to point out that these theoretical implications could not be derived from the ordinary approaches to vocabulary measurement.

A word may be entered in passing about the theoretical significance of the word-frequency variable, for that will prove to be the central concept in the pages that follow. Its importance rests on both empirical and theoretical grounds. Empirically, the word frequency has been found to obey a number of quantitative laws of great generality, like Zipf's law. It is therefore an extremely useful analytic tool. Theoretically, its importance derives from the fact that it represents the resultant of the many individual word choices that make up a person's speech. The central theoretical issues of language ultimately boil down to questions of how and why individual words are chosen in various situations. These individual acts of word selection are, of course, extremely difficult to control experimentally, and theoretical propositions about the process of word selection are often best tested experimentally by examining their consequences for repeated choices and testing these theorems against observed word frequencies. This is the basis on which rest most of the mathematical theories of Zipf's law and the other laws governing the word frequency.

When applied to the language produced by aphasic patients, Zipf's law opens up new possibilities of interpretation that do not exist under the ordinary vocabulary measures. Suppose, for example, we find that in aphasia the mathematical form of the equation for the word-frequency distribution is altered. That result would indicate that the dynamics of the process by which words are selected are altered by the brain lesion. If, on the other hand, aphasic language is found to conform to the equation for normal language, we may reasonably infer that the dynamics of the word-selection process have not been disturbed.

In actual fact, we have found that the law does hold for the language of aphasics. We may then compare the parameters of the equation for the patients with their values for normals. For all but the mildest cases there is, in fact, a characteristic shift of parameter values. The change in parameter values provides a complete and theoretically meaningful measure of the way in which the vocabulary distribution of the patient has changed as a consequence of the aphasia. Since the log-normal equation contains two parameters, the existence of Zipf's law allows us to represent the patient's word-frequency distribution by only two numbers.

We have by no means exhausted the list of benefits to be gained by approaching the vocabulary question in this way. The interrelations between the two parameters and other measurable properties of aphasic speech can add important information. The average rate at which a patient speaks provides a good example. Most patients, if fairly severely disturbed, speak at a rate well below the normal range. Certain patients, however, those with jargon, tend to speak at a rate equal to or even greater than the normal. Yet both types of patient show a similar vocabulary change, as measured by the change in the parameters of Zipf's law. If one were only to listen to the jargon patient, one might well conclude that the jargon patient's vocabulary had not been affected by the lesion, because with his increased output more different words appear in a given period of time. The pattern of measurements of verbal production, of which the word-frequency distribution is only part, thus gives us an objective basis for defining different types of aphasic disorder.

I do not want to leave the impression that all problems of measurement and interpretation disappear with the use of a quantitative analysis of this kind. On the contrary, many new ones arise. But these problems take us beyond the mere question of vocabulary size and provide us with deeper insights into the processes by which vocabulary is generated.

II

Compared with aphasia, word blindness presents some features that facilitate quantitative analysis and others that render it more difficult. The character of the basic deficit is much more clearly delimited than in aphasia. As it happens, moreover, this specific deficit is nicely suited to analysis with experimental methods that have been worked out for normal subjects. On the other hand, reception of language is always more difficult to study objectively than its emission. And in the study of word blindness we are forced to compare the patient's inability to perceive written words with his perception of nonverbal visual stimuli, while in aphasia we can go a long way by studying the patient's surviving language relative only to normal language. Though it may come as a surprise to those who regard visual perception as a thoroughly studied field, our study of word blindness is more seriously limited by gaps in our knowledge of the visual perception of objects than of the perception of verbal materials.

In the analysis of word blindness, as with aphasia, we are fortunate in being able to study the central defect by means of an experiment governed by a known empirical law. The experiment is the perception of words from single brief visual presentations. Seventy-five years ago McKeen Cattell (1885) showed that the perception span for familiar words in normal subjects is nearly as great as it is for single letters exposed for the same duration. That is, a normal person can perceive about four times as many letters from a flash of given duration if they are organized into common words as when they are arranged in isolation or in random sequences.

The Cattell effect gives us a good experimental definition of precisely the function that is defective in cases of word blindness. In severe cases, of course, the perception of individual letters may also be defective. But the central and striking defect is the patient's relative inability to see words in contrast to letters. This is exactly opposite to the striking feature of Cattell's effect: the normal person's relative inability to see letters in contrast to words.

Quantitative analysis of the Cattell effect became possible when it was shown that the duration threshold of a written word (i.e., the duration for which the word must be presented in order to be identified correctly) is proportional to the frequency of that word in general linguistic usage (Howes and Solomon [1951]). Figure 2 presents in graphical form the mathematical relationships as they have recently been worked out (Howes [1962]). The ordinate shows the duration of the visual exposure, the abscissa shows the frequency of occurrence of the word on a logarithmic scale. The different sets of data are for different threshold criteria: the top line (labeled $q = .9$) shows the duration for which words must be exposed in order to be perceived correctly on 90 per cent of exposures of that duration; the bottom set (labeled $q = .1$) on 10 per cent of exposures; and the central set (labeled $q = .5$) on 50 per cent of exposures, the usual criterion for a threshold. Notice that for every criterion value the threshold decreases in direct proportion to the logarithm of the word frequency. This relation extends over a range of nearly six logarithmic units, or a million to one in terms of word frequency. Note also that for rare or low-frequency words the curves for different threshold criteria show much greater dispersion than for common or high-frequency words. The characteristics of this dispersion have important theoretical implications in the same way that the mathematical form of Zipf's law does.

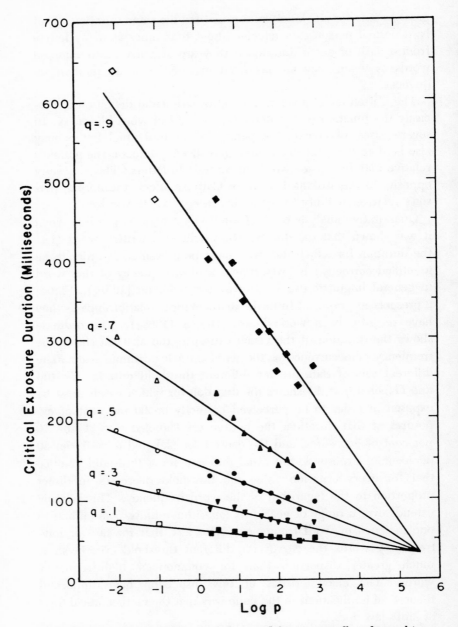

Figure 2.   Mathematical form of the word-frequency effect for tachisto-scopic perception of words. The abscissa gives the word frequency values (Lorge Magazine Count) in logarithmic units. The value of q specifies the probability with which a word of indicated frequency is correctly identified from an exposure of duration indicated by the ordinate.

The relationships shown in Figure 2 are fixed by only two constants, as was the case for Zipf's law. One represents the slope of the pivotal line, say the one for $q = .5$, and depends on such stimulus factors as the brightness of the flash, the size of the letters, etc. The other constant determines the spacing of the various lines for different criteria. (It does not, however, affect the relative spacing of lines—i.e., the fact that the lines for low-probability criteria are more closely bunched than those for high criteria—which is a characteristic of the equation itself.) Only two numbers, then, are needed to give a complete description of the word-perception process.

In principle we should be able to proceed to analyze the word perception of dyslexic patients much as we did the vocabulary of aphasics. In practice, however, many more complications arise with this experimental technique than with the word-frequency distributions. Resolving them will be neither easy nor quick.

Let me mention a few. For one thing, the Cattell effect seems large when looked at in terms of differences between extreme cases (e.g., nonsense syllables versus very common words). But for purposes of quantitative analysis the magnitude of the effect is rather small. Threshold variability for individual words is correspondingly large. This variability is to be expected, since lability is a fundamental characteristic of the human language process, and therefore is of no particular theoretical significance. But it does create a number of practical obstacles to experimentation.

To determine the equation of Figure 2 we must measure the probability of perception for each test word at each of many different exposure durations. To do this we would like to give repeated exposures of the same word to the same subject. But once the subject has seen the word, his expectation on subsequent exposures is greatly increased and the threshold of the word consequently decreased. Hence we can use a word only once in a given experimental session. There are ways of getting around this difficulty: by adopting an ascending psychophysical method, by averaging across comparable subjects or across different words of the same frequency of occurrence. The data shown in Figure 2, for instance, **are averages** based on twenty subjects. The data for individual subjects, though they show the same general relationships, are degraded too much by variability to permit a quantitative evaluation of parameter values. If we are to study word blindness with these methods, however, we cannot average the data from different patients, whose reading defects may be due to different lesions or at least to similar lesions of different degrees of severity. Hence we must find a way of generating data as clear as those of Figure 2 from a single experimental subject. We are currently working on several approaches to this goal, but, though we have made some progress, we are still far from achieving it.

Another complication is the right homonymous hemianopia that characteristically appears in certain types of word blindness. One can attempt to circumvent this difficulty by using short words, which do not extend into the bad field, by shifting the patient's fixation point into the good field, or by projecting words vertically instead of horizontally. Each solution, however, introduces its own problems, and again we have not yet achieved a fully satisfactory procedure.

Still another difficulty, and perhaps the thorniest, is that nothing comparable to the word-frequency effect has been worked out for the perception of nonverbal stimuli. Analogies certainly exist— familiar faces are seen with less exposure than unfamiliar ones, for example—but no method of quantifying such effects has ever been suggested. Precious little, in fact, even in a qualitative way, has been done with the effect of familiarization on the perception of objects. It is a curious lacuna in the field of perception. Yet in the most interesting cases of word blindness, those with an isolated defect, we particularly want to know whether or not there is any analogous dysfunction of perception for nonverbal stimuli. This question is of added interest because of its bearing on the type of mechanism for word blindness discussed by Dr. Geschwind, and I shall return to it at the end of my discussion.

III

Let me now describe our initial results. The patient, Mr. H., is a highly skilled artisan 65 years old. Though he had only five years of formal schooling, he worked successively as a watchmaker and in skilled jobs in electronic plants. There is no doubt that before his disease he was able to read very well. In the type of work in which he was engaged his vision obviously had to be excellent. Of the clinical findings upon his admission to the hospital, we need note here only the presence of the right homonymous hemianopia typically found in these cases. It did not spare the macula. Speech and writing were normal. Visual acuity, tested with the Snellen chart, was 20/20 in one eye and 20/40 in the other (with spectacles). The patient had no discernible difficulty recognizing people or objects even in the earlier stages of the disease, though he did have difficulty in identifying the colors of objects.

This difficulty with colors, by the way, is quite striking and has some very curious characteristics. Though reported in a number of previous cases of this type of word blindness, it has never been adequately described and studied, perhaps because one of its outstanding characteristics seems to be its variability. In our patient the defect was highly erratic. When it appeared it was usually extreme. The patient would not be able to identify the color of a wide sash of bright red, for example, yet he would occasionally surprise by naming correctly a color of much smaller expanse in the next minute. There seemed to be no rhyme or reason either to the correct identifications or the errors. The difficulty did not appear to be confined to particular hues; indeed, the patient even would report hues where there were none, as in calling a pitcher of milk in a picture yellow and identifying it as orange juice instead of milk. Often the patient seemed strangely vague when trying to name the color of an object, though seldom did he report that a colored object was colorless (i.e., gray, black or white). Before we were able to study this color defect further it quite suddenly cleared up, after having remained more or less stable for months. It would have been particularly interesting to investigate the patient's ability to match colors even when he misnamed them. Whether this difficulty with colors is functionally related to word blindness, or is only accidentally associated with it, we of course have no way of knowing. But its persistent occurrence in conjunction with what is otherwise such an isolated disorder is certainly striking. The statistical character of the color difficulty, moreover, its fluctuation from minute to minute, has certain parallels in the patient's reading defect.

Our experiments with this patient consisted of determining rough thresholds for a series of printed words and a series of objects. The ascending method of limits was used throughout: that is, the stimulus was shown first at a level well below the level at which it could be seen and was gradually increased on successive exposures until perceived. The apparatus was a slide projector equipped with camera shutter for tachistoscopic control and Wratten neutral-density filters for intensity control. In these exploratory studies we varied both intensity and duration, in order to see if they had differential effects on the patient's word perception, although it is generally more satisfactory to hold the intensity constant and vary only the duration. The slides of words were prepared by photographing words carefully printed on special paper to obtain very good contrast.

The experimental words were selected to cover the range of word frequencies determined by the Lorge Magazine Count of four and a half million words at each of three lengths; three, seven, and eleven letters. Arabic and Roman numerals were added. Selection of objects for the control study of nonverbal perception presented a more difficult problem, since there is no theoretical rule to follow. We chose a set of line drawings by well-known artists from the files of local art galleries. In this way we can take advantage of a convenient system for designating and reproducing the exact drawings in different laboratories. The largest number of these drawings depict animals (e.g., dog, rabbit, horse, monkey, camel). Others represent people in various situations (e.g., a woman praying, two men drinking, four people sitting on a bench). All are drawn in clear black lines of high contrast. A single exception was Stuart's unfinished portrait of Washington, which we included in order to have a very familiar face in the series. Each picture could be identified by a simple description, usually by a name. To these drawings of objects we added some line drawings of simple geometric figures (e.g., triangle, star, etc.).

In any one experimental session with the patient we are of course able to present only a few of these slides. Some of them have not yet been used with the patient, whom we examine only once a month. The attempt to identify words is extremely fatiguing—and discouraging as well—to the patient, as are his efforts to read ordinary text.

The ascending series of tachistoscopic presentations changed both in intensity and in duration, starting with 1/10 second exposure at the lowest intensity. The intensity was then increased gradually through three logarithmic units, after which the duration was lengthened to 1/5 second and the intensity returned to the lowest value. The intensity was then increased again through three logarithmic units, whereupon the duration was lengthened to 1/2 second, etc. Since intensity and duration of exposure are not reciprocally related in this range, a two-dimensional display is needed for these data. In Figure 3 the arrow describes the path of

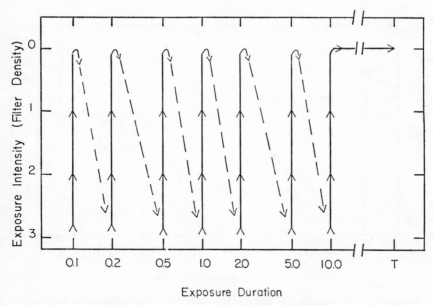

Figure 3. Ascending series of tachistoscopic exposures used in determining word thresholds. Duration is in seconds; T indicates a continuous time exposure.

the regular ascending series. We did not present the stimulus at every possible combination of intensity and duration, of course, but skipped through the series according to our judgment of the expected threshold as indicated by previous measurements. In addition to two normal control subjects who were tested separately, one person from our staff viewed the stimulus presentations at the same time as the patient and thus served as an additional informal control. We plan to study a hemianopic patient without word blindness as a separate control, but have not yet had such a patient available for testing.

The results for three-letter words are shown in Figure 4. Solid figures are for the patient, open ones for one control subject. With the normal it was never necessary to go beyond exposures of one tenth of a second; with the patient it was necessary to proceed to longer exposure durations (i.e., more than two logarithmic units of intensity above the thresholds of the control subject) for more

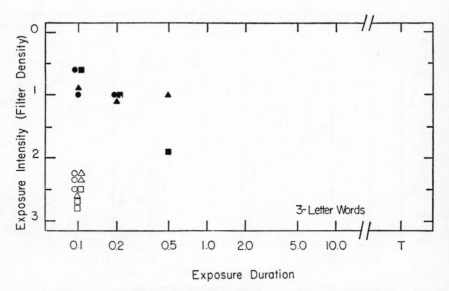

Figure 4. Thresholds for three-letter words. Co-ordinates as in Figure 3. Open figures: normal control subject. Filled figures: Word-blind patient. Squares, circles, and triangles indicate words of high, medium, and low frequency, respectively.

than half the words. There is no overlap between the most difficult word for the normal and the easiest word for the patient.

A rough test of the word-frequency effect is indicated in Figure
4 by the different shapes of the data points. The three most frequent words are indicated by squares, the three medium-frequency
words by circles, and the three rarest words by triangles. For the
normal subject the data follow the word-frequency effect as expected: the two lowest thresholds are for common words, and two
of the three rare words have the highest thresholds. The rank-order
coefficient of correlation ρ is -0.50. For the patient, on the other
hand, no orderly progression from high-frequency words to low-frequency words is evident despite the tremendous range of intensities and durations that the data cover. In fact, the order of thresholds is perfectly random with respect to word frequency ($\rho =
+0.10$).

Figure 5 presents a similar graph for seven-letter words. The
control subject's thresholds are roughly the same as for three-letter

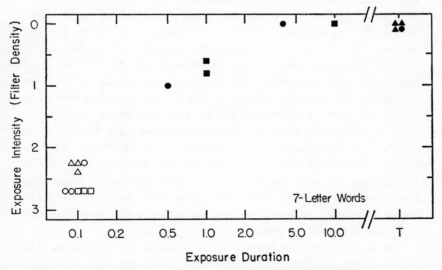

Figure 5.   Thresholds for seven-letter words. Co-ordinates as in Figure 3.
Open figures: normal control subject. Filled figures: Word-blind patient.
Squares, circles, and triangles indicate words of high, medium, and low
word frequency, respectively.

words, and again the word-frequency effect is evident. The patient's thresholds for these words are even higher than for three-letter words, the lowest threshold requiring that the exposure be increased to one half second. Though the word-frequency effect is again less in evidence in the patient's data than in the normal's, there is some indication of its presence in the fact that all three of the rare words have thresholds above the measurable range (i.e., with the shutter held open indefinitely). The data for eleven-letter words (not shown) resemble those for seven-letter words except that the differences are even more exaggerated. The patient's lowest threshold in this set of words required that the duration be raised to two seconds, and half of the words could not be correctly reported with exposures in the measurable range. There is again a slight indication of the word-frequency effect, as the rarest eleven-letter words were all among those identified only with exposures beyond the measurable range.

It would be foolish to draw any conclusions from so few data. But let me enter one or two comments on these results as though they were confirmed by data on many words. It is worth mentioning first of all that measuring thresholds of words for this patient is a feasible task, something not altogether self-evident in the case of this patient before the experiment was tried. The word blindness, moreover, especially for three-letter words, is far from complete. The much higher thresholds for seven- and eleven-letter words are perhaps accounted for by the hemianopia, though we wish to check this point by determining thresholds for the same words on a hemianopic patient without word blindness. The accuracy with which word thresholds can be determined appears to be adequate for following the course of recovery and for comparing the extent of the disorder in different patients. In short, the technique, even with all the imperfections noted in the preceding section, is able to produce results.

The most interesting feature of the data is the suggestion that the word-frequency equation does not hold for three-letter words.[1]

---

[1] In a somewhat similar patient, Professor H.-L. Teuber (personal communication) has observed that the patient's errors on a standard reading test were unrelated to word frequency. Though the task is admittedly quite a different one from that of determination of word thresholds, his observations represent an interesting parallel to our own preliminary finding.

This is in contrast to our finding for vocabulary changes in aphasia. There, if you recall, the equation for the Zipf law retains its mathematical form even in the most severely affected patients we have studied; only the constants of the equation are changed. Hence our conclusion that in aphasia the fundamental linguistic process that generates the vocabulary distribution is not disturbed, and the vocabulary disturbance consequently is of a quantitative rather than a qualitative nature. The results for our case of word blindness—assuming that it holds up under further experimentation—indicates, to the contrary, that the process that generates the word-frequency effect is itself inoperative since the equation no longer holds. This fits well the interpretation of the case defended by Dr. Geschwind: for if the language areas of the brain, which from the evidence of aphasia we may suppose to be the source of word-frequency information, are disconnected from the visual areas, it is hard to see how the word-frequency effect on perception could operate.

The correlation between word frequency and the thresholds of seven- and eleven-letter words may seem to conflict with the result for three-letter words. But it is more likely that these correlations simply reflect the fact that words as long as that extend far enough into the patient's defective visual field that their right-hand portions are effectively blotted out. The patient therefore is forced to guess at their completions, and naturally guesses the more familiar words first. Several details of the threshold data support this view; study of control subjects with hemianopias but without word blindness will provide an additional method of testing the issue. This completion or guessing effect does not generate the same mathematical relationship between threshold and word-frequency as the word-frequency effect proper (Howes [1962]), and accurate experimental determination of the form of the function can distinguish between them. Because of the complication introduced by the right hemianopia when long words are used, the data obtained with short words are of much greater significance for the study of word perception.

Let us turn to the data for object perception, which are shown in Figure 6. For the normal subject these thresholds are generally higher than his word thresholds. With the patient, on the other hand, they are about equal to his thresholds for three-letter words

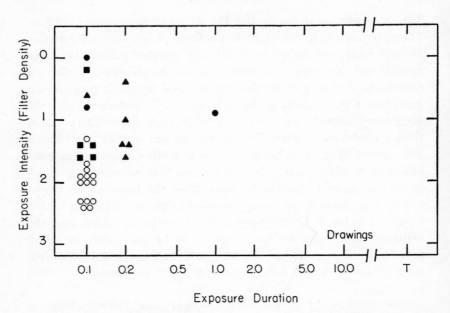

Figure 6. Thresholds for drawings. Co-ordinates as in Figure 3. Open figures: normal control subject. Solid figures: word-blind patient. Squares, circles, and triangles indicate drawings of low, medium, and high threshold for the control subject.

and much lower than those for seven- or eleven-letter words. On the average, the patient's thresholds for objects are higher than the normal's, though the difference is less than for three-letter words and there is considerable overlap between the patient's lowest object thresholds and the normal's highest. At least part of the difference may, of course, be accounted for by the patient's hemianopia.

Nothing comparable to the word-frequency equation is known for object perception. We can, however, at least determine whether or not the patient's thresholds for different objects follow the same order as the normal's thresholds. Insofar as object thresholds in normals obey a principle analogous to the word-frequency effect, this comparison will tell us whether the patient follows the same principle. In Figure 6 the patient's thresholds for the pictures with the lowest, medium, and highest thresholds for the normal subject are represented by different symbols (square, circle, and triangle, respectively), and we can see that the patient's thresholds correspond very closely to their order for the normal subject. There is, however, a distinct indication of increased variability in the patient's perceptual performance, a trait mentioned before in connection with his color vision.

Our preliminary findings on this patient thus indicate that object perception is not completely spared, as one might have adjudged from clinical examination, though it is much less affected than word perception. Though the word-frequency effect appears to be abolished, in object perception the order of perceptual difficulty found in the normal is retained in the patient. This, of course, may only reflect differences of intrinsic perceptual difficulty between the various pictures rather than any effect of their relative familiarity in the analogy to the word-frequency effect.

The significance of these findings is illuminated by a brief comparison with the results from a second patient with word blindness but without right hemianopia and with agraphia. This patient also fails to show the word-frequency effect, but for a different reason. Though he clearly understands the instructions, the patient is practically never able to say the word that is presented even when he can easily spell out all the letters. Having spelled the word *pet* correctly as *p-e-t*, for example, he hesitated when asked to say the word and finally came out with *place*. He has the same difficulty when the word is spelled orally to him. Obviously, the concept of a word threshold has no real meaning in this case. Yet the patient's perception of letters is quite normal, and the levels at which he is able to spell a stimulus word correctly are roughly the same as those at which a normal subject can identify a random series of letters that does not form a word. Thresholds for pictures of objects show no trace of a deficit, his identifications being extremely quick and accurate. The patient's conversational speech is good, and vocabulary as measured by the word-frequency distribution is normal. He easily repeats any word on command, even rare or long ones, despite his inability to find even a short word when it is spelled to him.

This patient's word blindness would seem to be a consequence of a very specific and nearly total spelling defect. Under ordinary circumstances loss of the ability to spell does not interfere with the ability to hear, understand, and produce spoken language, but it makes the reading of an alphabetic script impossible. Hence the disorder in this second case is not really a visual disturbance, but only appears that way because reading and writing are the most important functions that depend on spelling ability.

Because the disorder appears to be so specific to the spelling function, and since the patient shows no difficulty whatever in verbally identifying drawings, one might hope that he could be trained to read words as ideographs rather than alphabetically. On this point one naturally looks for clarification to a language like Japanese, which commonly uses both alphabetic and ideographic scripts. But what little I have been able to find on word blindness in that language (Panse and Shimoyama [1955]) is not clearly enough described to be useful. A case of word blindness in a Chinese financier who spoke both English and Chinese fluently has, however, been carefully described by Lyman, Kwan, and Chao (1938). In this case, which generally resembles our second patient, both reading and writing were about equally affected in the two languages. Their finding rather surprises us. Why a patient who can identify drawings perfectly[2] should be unable to name ideographs perfectly is hard to understand. It certainly goes against the otherwise clear picture of an isolated spelling defect provided by our case. We need to know much more about the process of ideographic reading and about the role of spelling in alphabetically written languages (which may not be quite so simple as it seems at first glance) before we can understand the nature of the reading disorder in these patients (see Money's discussion of directional orientation, above, p. 21). Certainly a careful study of word-blind patients in a language like Japanese, which

---

[2] Actually, Lyman *et al.* do not report any *specific* testing of their patient's ability to name and recognize objects. In view of the detail with which their examination was otherwise conducted, we presume that they detected no indication of any disturbance of these functions. Our own patient of this type showed none even under the kind of tachistoscopic examination that revealed a mild disturbance in our first patient.

would permit regular comparison between ideographic and alphabetic writing (see section on other languages by Money), would be of extreme value in this connection.

The word blindness in our two patients evidently represents two quite different disorders, despite the fact that there is a loss of the word-frequency relationship in both cases. The absence of right hemianopia in the second case rules out the mechanism for word blindness described by Dr. Geschwind, which seems to fit the first case so well. Thus even when the patients do not differ in regard to the basic relationship under investigation, the experimental methods are capable of discrimination between different patterns of breakdown.

Let me emphasize once again that the interpretations I have discussed here are admittedly based on insufficient data. Further data may modify or even reverse some of these initial results. It is the method of studying these cases, more than the present data, that I think is worth calling to your attention. Tachistoscopic study of neurological cases is nothing new, of course. My point here has been to illustrate the added power, both for descriptive and interpretive purposes, that is to be gained by an analysis based on a quantitative law that governs the data produced by the tachistoscopic technique.

IV

Let us return now to the theory of the lesion producing word blindness discussed by Dr. Geschwind. The mechanism he proposed attributes word blindness to the joint occurrence of two lesions: one destroying the left visual cortex and the second destroying the splenium and perhaps adjoining white matter of the left occipital cortex. The patient is word blind because his left visual cortex is incapable of receiving visual information and his right visual cortex, which receives visual information normally, is unable to communicate with the language areas in the left cortex. The crux of the theory is the assumption that the visual pattern that constitutes a word physically cannot be processed into a word *as a whole* and labeled, identified, recognized—whatever you want to call it—because it is cut off from the language areas. It rests, then, on a distinction between what goes on in the healthy right visual cortex when one presents the patient with a written word and the finished process of word perception, which requires further processing by the language areas.

The attraction of this mechanism is that it obviates the need for inventing a special center in the left occipital lobe whose function is the perception of words in contradistinction to all other visual stimuli. By attributing the selective disturbance of visual language to the independently established facts of the laterality of the speech areas on the one hand and the hemianopia on the other, the disconnection mechanism achieves greater elegance and parsimony than the hypothesis of a special center.

On closer examination, as Dr. Geschwind has mentioned, the disconnection hypothesis runs into difficulty. If, indeed, the visual areas in the right occipital cortex are isolated from the language areas, how is the patient able to name *objects* presented to him visually? Should not the disconnection between the visual and language areas also interrupt this function? Reading a word, after all, consists of finding the right word for a specific visual pattern. Is not naming an object or the drawing of an object essentially the same process?

One basis for an explanation of this difference is that objects, unlike written scripts, are palpable. Visual information from objects may therefore be communicated to the somatosensory areas in the right (ipsilateral) hemisphere and from there could communicate with the language areas in the left hemisphere through the intact portion of the corpus callosum served by the anterior cerebral artery. This type of explanation implies a *rerouting* of visual information about objects that is forbidden to writing. It depends on the existence of a mechanism for the transfer of perceptual information from the visual areas to the somatosensory areas analogous to the transfer that Sperry (1961) has shown to exist between the right and left visual areas.

The main difficulty with this type of explanation is in understanding why visual information about written script should be excluded from the visuotactile transfer process. True, the most striking examples of visuotactile coordination involve the palpation of objects under visual examination. But when we write, some coordination of tactile or kinesthetic information about letters with their visual form is surely required. Since the evidence indicates that visuotactile transfer for objects must be built up by experience (Hebb, 1949), should not this experience with visuotactile coordination of written forms also result in their transfer? Perhaps the fact that the cases cited by Dr. Geschwind are right-handed provides a key. In a right-handed writer, visuotactile transfer for writing might be built up in the left hemisphere but not in the right hemisphere, where the coordination involved in the act of writing does not take place. That bilateral (interhemispherical) transfer of language between the somatosensory areas would be inconsiderable follows from the fact that writing with the left hand is nearly always very poor for a right-handed person. Consequently, in the patients we are considering, there exists a basis in the right hemisphere for a rerouting of visual information about objects to the language areas but not for visual information about writing. The explanation may seem a bit forced, but it is this kind of detailed analysis that is required to take into account all the facts of these cases.

A second way of accounting for a word-blind patient's ability to name visually-presented objects is to assume that the disconnection between the visual and language areas is incomplete and that the surviving tracts are adequate to transmit information about objects but not about written words. The fibers connecting the two areas are considered to be equipotential for visual information, whether it be from objects or from written language. This second type of explanation treats the functional difference between verbal and nonverbal visual stimuli as basically quantitative rather than qualitative, and is thus akin to Lashley's principle (1929) of *mass action* in brain function.

At first glance, the assumption that more extensive tracts are required for the transmission of visual information about words than about visual objects may appear paradoxical. Are not words much simpler as visual stimuli than line drawings of objects or than objects themselves? With loss of all but a small amount of the connections between the visual and language areas, would not the simpler word stimuli be passed and the more complex object stimuli rejected—exactly the opposite of what is found in the clinical picture? The paradox rests on the implicit inference that because pictures of objects are more complex than words *physically* they are also more complex from the viewpoint of brain function. And that does not necessarily follow.

We find ourselves here in the midst of a problem that has never, to my knowledge, been analyzed adequately: the relation of the relative difficulty of different behavioral tasks to the principle of mass action. Lashley left the problem with the simple rule, based on the special case of maze learning, that more difficult tasks show greater deficit from lesions of given size. But that rule is too simple to be useful in evaluating the relative difficulty of reading versus the verbal identification of visually presented objects.

Let us compare the two tasks first with regard to how difficult they are to learn. Learning to read is one of the most difficult perceptual tasks human beings are called on to perform. To master the task of reading, children require arduous practice for many years, long after object-naming is highly developed. On this basis we should argue that reading is the more difficult task. Then, if we extend Lashley's rule, reading ought also to be the function more severely disturbed by a given amount of neural destruction.

Once a person has learned to read, however, the comparison changes. As we have seen, thresholds for printed words are generally lower than thresholds for pictures or simple geometric forms. Similarly, the latency of association to words is much shorter than to the corresponding objects or line drawings of them (Karwoski, Gramlich, and Arnott [1944]). The task of reading, once acquired, would thus seem to be less difficult than object-naming.

The contradiction can be resolved if we consider that transmission of visual information about written words may require more equipotential neural tissue connecting the visual and language areas than is required for visual objects. While reading is being learned, more neural tissue must be brought under the functional control of this class of visual stimuli and consequently the learning task is more difficult in the sense that it requires more time and practice. Once the learning is completed, however, the larger proportion of tissue used in the reading act provides for lower thresholds and shorter latencies, as is usual in nerve-trunk functions. Partial sectioning of these tracts would therefore severely cripple reading while producing only a relatively slight disturbance of object-naming.

Some testable consequences follow from this line of interpretation. Object perception should be at least slightly disturbed in word blindness of the kind we are considering. We have seen that tachistoscopic study of our patient supports this consequence by demonstrating that object-naming is not undisturbed, in contrast with the second patient whose word blindness is not due to disconnection. Moreover, one would expect that those patients whose word perception is more severely affected will also be those whose object perception is worse. This assertion can be tested by comparing both different patients and the same patients at different stages in the evolution of the disorder.

The perplexing functional distinction between objects and words as visual stimuli in these cases of word blindness calls to mind one other line of evidence suggesting a parallel distinction. This evidence comes from the Innsbruck investigations on reversal of the visual world by means of prisms (Kohler [1951]). When the subject first puts on the prisms he perceives the world as reversed. He then gradually learns to compensate for the reversal in his actions, until he is so skilled that the casual observer watching him would assume his vision to be normal. Yet the subject still reports that he sees his visual world as reversed: automobiles, for example, appear to him to drive down the left side of the road, even though he behaves as if they are on the right. When the subject has worn the prisms for a very long time—many weeks or months—his visual world may return to normal; that is, the visual world reverses itself so that automobiles now appear to drive down the right side of the street even when viewed through the reversing prisms. This reversal does not seem to occur piecemeal, nor is the subject aware that it is occurring; rather, he just suddenly realizes at some moment that it has taken place.

Now a very interesting observation has been reported in this connection. When this reversal occurs it affects all objects in the visual world—trees, houses, people, etc.—with one significant exception: writing often remains reversed. For example, automobiles will now appear on the right side of the street, but the numbers of their license plates are backwards. Similarly, a book held in the subject's right hand will appear to him as in his right hand rather than on his left, but the letters within the book remain reversed, and he has to read them by mirror reading. Written matter is the only class of visual stimuli that has been observed to show this independence of the remainder of the visual world.

These reversal studies, then, provide a second instance in which written matter appears to function as a special system of visual stimuli, distinct from all other objects in the visual world. The separation reported in these experiments may be quite unrelated to the functional separation of writing and visual objects in cases of word blindness, of course. Yet it is tempting to look for a common mechanism. In terms of the mass-action principle, for instance, one could argue that the difference results from the fact that written language is a much more difficult class of visual stimuli for the brain to learn to process than any other class of visual stimuli. Just as it takes much longer for the child to learn how to handle written material in learning to read, so it requires more experience for the adult wearing reversing prisms to relearn how to handle written forms than it does for any other class of visual stimuli.

V

Though my remarks in this paper have been confined to the problem of word blindness as it exists in adults with brain disease, much of what I have had to say has, I believe, some useful application to the developmental dyslexias as well. I am aware, of course, that the latter types of cases may result from very different causes. Yet if satisfactory quantitative methods, both experimental and conceptual, can be developed for analyzing the basic disturbances of language that are involved in the reading process in any one form of dyslexia, I believe those methods will prove generally useful in other forms. For the field is still at a stage where we need to find out exactly what dyslexia is as well as why it occurs.

10

Dyslexia and the Maturation of Visual Function

HERBERT G. BIRCH

In preparing this paper, a choice had to be made between the path of presenting a body of data stemming from research on the problem of reading disability in children and that of sharing with the group the kinds of thinking and theoretical considerations that underlay the development of the investigations themselves. The latter course has been chosen because of the conviction that unless we explore our fundamental approaches to a problem as complex as the one we have under scrutiny, the details of our findings may frequently obscure the broad lines of inquiry we are pursuing, the fundamental hypotheses which are being explored, and so come to be viewed as mere additional facts rather than as stimuli and provocations for renewed and more intensive study.

At the outset it is necessary to point out that dyslexia is not in itself a problem capable of being investigated. Rather, as has been so fully demonstrated in the work of Rabinovitch and others who have studied disturbances in samples of children who have exhibited reading disabilities, it represents a disturbance of functional product which may derive from a variety of etiologies. Heterogeneity of associated disorders rather than any single disturbance has tended to characterize the group. Given a complex disturbance which may stem from so diverse a series of antecedents as personality disorder, neurological damage, and cultural deprivation, it is necessary for any investigator to make certain strategic decisions as to the aspect of the problem he wishes to explore before it is possible to develop a meaningful program of systematic inquiry. It is most important to recognize that when such a strategic choice has been made, it in no way indicates that the investigator does not believe that factors other than the ones which he himself has chosen for study are unimportant in the production of the functional disturbance. Therefore, in having selected the problem of the maturation of visual function as the region for my own exploration, I have in no way been guided by the view that factors other than the ones with which I happen to be concerned are either irrelevant or unimportant in some cases of reading disturbance.

The elaboration and the choice of a research strategy stems not only from analysis of what may be an important set of mechanisms in the development of a disturbed pattern of behavior, but also from the background of experience of the investigator. The scientist's personal history functions to determine the kinds of thoughts he may have about a problem and the techniques which he can begin to use to approach it. Just as the occupational biases of the psychiatrist turn him to a consideration of problems of motivation and personality organization, and those of the sociologist to a consideration of environmental and subcultural variables, my own background as a comparative psychologist and as a student of human development leads me to a consideration of the nature of the perceptual demands which may underlie the development of reading skills, and to a concern with the kinds of developmental regulations which are necessary for their acquisition.

Two concepts in comparative psychology are of special value in helping us to develop an approach to some of the disordered mechanisms which may underlie reading disability. The first of these is the view that one of the ways in which organisms differ from one another is in the hierarchical organization of their sensory systems. Thus, various animals belonging to the same class exhibit characteristically different patterns of behavior as a consequence of the sensory systems which are predominant in the organization of their responsiveness. As every good fisherman knows before he baits his hook, different fish are characterized by the degree to which olfactory, gustatory or visual aspects of the environment are primarily determinative in the development of their responses. In addition, among mammalian forms, breeds of dogs and the practices which are most effective in their training are dependent to a very large extent upon whether the dog is one in whom smell or vision is the hierarchically predominant sense modality. In an animal in whom vision represents the predominant sense mode, the other avenues of sensory input are utilized as background information which is integrated around the pre-eminent visual stimulus. However, in organisms in which another sensory modality is the primary hierarchically positioned avenue of information, visual stimulation becomes part of the background and is not the primarily determinative avenue through which behavior is organized. The hierarchical organization of sensory systems, therefore, functions to a very large extent to determine which aspects of the environment constitute figure and which aspects constitute background.

As soon as one begins to apply the concept of sensory-system hierarchy to the human developmental process, it becomes apparent that the developing child goes through a number of sequences in the course of which alterations in the nature of the hierarchical structuring of avenues of sense occur. In the young infant interoceptive sensory modalities and visceral sensations are predominant. Stimulation of the visual or of the auditory system is only of secondary importance and constitutes background rather than figure in the organization of the response. In the normal individual, in the course of time the teleoreceptor systems come to dominate over visceral and proximal reception until complex patterning of behavior comes to be pre-eminently organized around information derived from the teleoreceptor systems of audition and vision. The sequence of change is beautifully illustrated in the series of studies by Renshaw and his associates (1930) on body surface localization. In the young child visual information serves to interfere with the accuracy of localization of touched points on the

body surface whereas, in the older child and adult, visual information facilitates and makes more accurate the location of previous
tactual stimulation.

One hypothesis concerning the genesis of some kinds of reading
disability stems immediately from this view of both comparative
psychology and of the developmental sequence. One can postulate
that reading disability may stem from the inadequate development
of appropriate hierarchical organization of sensory systems and so,
at least in part, be the product of the failure of visual system
hierarchical dominance. In such cases, concurrent stimulation in
sensory modalities such as the visceral or proprioceptive will function not as essential background to the organization of the visual
percept but as a displacement stimulus resulting in the disorganiza-
tion of visual response and the appropriation of the visual stimulation to the nonvisual pattern of arousal and behavioral organization.
It is clear that, from this point of view, one of the essential features
in the development of so-called reading readiness is the organization of a hierarchical set of relations among the sensory systems
wherein the teleoreceptor systems, particularly the visual, become
hierarchically dominant. Failure for such dominance to occur will
result in a pattern of functioning which is inappropriate for the
development of reading skill.

With this hypothesis in mind, my colleagues and I have begun
to explore the organization of hierarchical relations among sense
systems in the child. The model which we have chosen is a simple
two-window discrimination learning situation in which the making
of a correct choice is rewarded by the obtaining of a chocolate-
covered raisin. The child is seated in front of an apparatus containing two windows side by side. If the correct choice is made
when the child lifts the cover, he will find a reward which he may
take and eat, or keep. The learning task involves the recognition
that the window containing the reward is that one which is on the
same side as that to which a stimulus has been applied. Thus, if
a child is touched on his right arm, it is the window on that side
behind which the reward will be located. If he is touched on his
left, that then represents the side that is baited. Similarly, if
his chair is tilted to the right or to the left, the directional tilt

will determine the correctness of choice. In such a situation, the child may be stimulated by sound, light, touch, or displacement of his position in space.

When such a learning situation is used, a first measure of hierarchical dominance may be obtained in terms of the identification of that sensory system which is first learned when a mixed-modalities presentation of stimulation is used. Thus in any sequence of twenty trials, five of the signals given will be in the visual, five in the auditory, five in the tactual, and five in the spatial displacement modality. Separate learning curves are then plotted for each of the modalities. The number of trials required for the acquisition of the correct responses to a predetermined criterion of learning, then, can provide a first order indication of the sense system to which the child is most readily responsive in his learning, as well as the more general hierarchical ordering.

A second method for the exploration of hierarchical dominance among the sense avenues is permitted through the use of a conflict model. In this model the child is permitted to learn the correct response up to a criterion in each of the modalities that is being explored. Once equivalent levels of acquisition have been achieved for each of the modalities, conflicting information of a bimodal kind is presented. Thus, a sound is presented on the right simultaneously with a tactual stimulation on the left; or a visual flash on the left by a tilting of the chair to the right. The choices made by the child then reflect the sense avenues to which he is pre-eminently responsive in the organization of his choice behavior.

Thus far, in the use of these models only preliminary data are available. However, even at this point, it is possible to state that marked individual differences exist in the sense systems which dominate in the organization of the behaviors studied. From the point of view of the hypothesis under consideration, it should be possible to isolate and identify a group among children with reading disability who are different from normal learners because they have a different hierarchical organization of their avenues of sense. Further, from a developmental point of view, it would be expected that with age, the teleoreceptive systems would come to be increasingly dominant over the proximal receptive avenues of information. Both these problems are at present being explored.

A second general avenue of approach to the problem of reading disability is suggested by the view in comparative psychology that the evolution of behavior can be conceptualized as the process of the development of intersensory patterning. As Sir Charles Sherrington (1951) has pointed out, the essential strategy in the evolution of the central nervous system has been not the elaboration of new avenues of sense, but rather the development of increased liaison among the existent major sensory input systems. The unevenness of the development of such an intersensory liaison is illustrated nicely by the behavior of the frog. As long ago as 1882, the naturalist-physician Abbott demonstrated that the frog was incapable of modifying a visually determined response on the basis of information obtained through pain sensation. Thus, a frog who was permitted to strike at a live fly impaled upon a central post which was surrounded by a sharp palisade of stakes continued to strike at the moving fly despite the fact that every outthrust of its tongue resulted in its being impaled upon the sharp points of the palisade. In Abbott's description, the visually determined striking response to the fly was continued even though the frog's tongue was ripped to shreds. Thus, no modulation of a visually-determined response occurred as a consequence of a tactual pain stimulus. In contrast, in the same organism, the visually-determined striking response is capable of being modified by information received through gustatory avenues of stimulation. Thus, as Schaeffer (Maier and Schneirla [1935], p. 213) has pointed out, a frog in very few trials will learn to inhibit its visually determined striking response to a hairy caterpillar; again in experiments in my own laboratories, the visually determined response to a moving target may be rapidly inhibited, when this target is coated with a bitter substance such as quinine. Therefore, in the frog, gustatory stimulation is capable of modulating and modifying visually-determined response whereas tactual stimulation is not. In contrast to the amphibian, in the normal mammal information deriving from all sense avenues may be adequately integrated and this liaison constitutes, perhaps, the major function of the cerebral cortex.

As Pavlov (1927) has pointed out, one of the first phenomena to be effected by damage to the central nervous system is the degree to which different sensory avenues may become equivalent one to the other. Whereas, in a normal mammal with an intact nervous system, visual stimulation readily can be conditioned to become equivalent to tactual or auditory stimulation, in the damaged organism, the development of such equivalences and their stability may be markedly disturbed. In addition, as Lashley (1929) has pointed out in his investigations, such phenomena as so-called conditional discrimination, wherein the capacity to distinguish between two relatively similar stimuli in a given modality is dependent upon the association with this stimulation of information provided in another modality, are among those most readily affected by damage to the central nervous system.

The analogical features and potential relations of these intersensory phenomena to the reading task are readily apparent. Reading, to be effective, requires the integration of visual information with information as to spatial direction and distribution. At a bare minimum it involves a sequence of visual experiences from left to right, and not merely an isolated visually-determined discrimination. In addition, in the reading of the English alphabet many of the discriminations among letters which take place are dependent upon the integration of the perceived visual *Gestalt* with spatially distributed information. Thus, such letters as b, p, d, and q all represent equivalent *Gestalten.* The distinction among them is dependent upon the degree to which the individual is capable of using positional information in association with the visual stimulus. It is equally apparent that such letters as N, and Z, or W and M bear similar relations one to the other.

One hypothesis which stems from the analysis of intersensory processes is that some individuals with reading disability are disabled precisely because they have nervous systems in which the development of equivalences between the sensory systems is impaired. The most obvious potential region of impairment would be between the visual and auditory systems, and one would predict that a greater number of children with reading disabilities would exhibit disturbances in the capacity to establish visual-auditory equivalences than would be found in a matched group drawn from the nondyslexic segment of the population. Similarly, it would be anticipated that the difficulties would not be limited to visual-auditory relationships, but would be extended to visual-kinesthetic and visual-tactual-kinesthetic relations as well. In our own researches, we have been primarily concerned with the problem of the degree to which a disordering in visual-tactual-kinesthetic relations may be present in children with reading disabilities. The model which we have used to explore this problem is one which employs geometrical forms to test a child's capacity to recognize and identify a tactual experience as being identical with a visual one, and a kinesthetic experience as being equivalent either to a tactual or visual experience. Thus far, our findings suggest that disturbances in visual-tactual and visual-kinesthetic relationships are far more frequent in the dyslexic segment of the population than among nondyslexic children.

The final concept guiding our researches that I should like to present derives from developmental psychology to a far greater extent than it does from comparative psychological considerations. For a number of years my colleagues and I have been deeply concerned with a tendency on the part of psychology increasingly to view perception as an essentially unitary event. Our explorations, particularly those conducted on both hemiplegic adults and neurologically damaged children by Bortner and myself (1960; 1962) have led us to the view that the phenomena of perception, when considered developmentally, lead to a concept of perceptual levels, which distinguishes an early level of perceptual discrimination from a later level of perceptual analysis and a still later level of perceptual synthesis. Thus, very young children are able to recognize objects and so discriminate between identities and nonidentities. This capacity is one which is least affected by neurological damage and is retained even by individuals who have sustained severe and serious traumata to the central nervous system. The second level which we have termed "perceptual analysis" consists of the capacity of the individual to separate out of a given *Gestalt,* the units of which this over-all figural organization is composed. This analytic capacity develops considerably later than does the capacity to make the recognition type of discrimination and is readily interfered with by central nervous system damage. Thus, neurologically damaged individuals quite capable of making clear-cut discriminations between different geometric forms may, however, be entirely incapable of choosing which of a number of strokes, lying at different angles, correctly matches the side of a test triangle. Similarly, individuals who are capable of discriminating between whole figures have great difficulty, in the presence of neurological damage, in distinguishing which one of a number of alternative groupings of unitary parts could effectively be combined to constitute a figural whole.

It is our hypothesis that one of the problems which contribute to the development of reading disability is the inadequate development of these higher and more complex levels of visual perceptual function. Thus, we would predict that among those with reading disability one could begin to identify cases in which markedly defective analytic and synthetic visual perceptual capacity exists. We are at present examining this hypothesis in normally and abnormally functioning school children.

It is clear that the three concepts with which we have dealt by no means encompass the wide variety of disturbances which may be identified in children with reading disability. However, they do represent a set of conceptualizations which derive from a particular theoretical approach to the evolution and development of behavioral functions. Consequently they focus our attention upon some aspects of the functional demands that reading makes upon the organism, and pose certain hypotheses as to the nature of some processes which may be interfered with in development and so result in a disturbance in functional product. The value of such an approach lies less in its universal explanatory character than in its value in providing ideas and directions for research. In our view it represents the explication of one aspect of the question which becomes experimentally manageable and which therefore permits of explorations in depth with the clear possibility of the identification of some mechanisms of disturbed functioning which may be important in the development of dyslexia.

11

Dyslexia in Relation to Diagnostic Methodology in Hearing and Speech Disorders

WILLIAM G. HARDY

On face value it would seem fruitful to explore some of the possible relations between clinical methods and findings applicable to hearing and speech problems and a general picture of dyslexia. To do this thoroughly is of course an impossible task for any one person.

Inasmuch as reading is a derived art and skill, in both developmental and linguistic terms, it is reasonable to expect to find some degree of reading disability associated with a wide variety of other communicative disorders. The facts seem to bear out this expectancy, although the documentation of the facts presently leaves much to be desired, largely, perhaps, because of the communicative gap between clinical and educative agencies. Various concepts and methods in fairly wide use by psychologists, audiologists, speech pathologists, and others concerned with the clinical assessment of language comprehension and use offer the possibility of more thorough documentation as time goes on.

In very general terms, the range of disorders in communication is usually described under one or another of four categories: hearing

171

impairment, speech deviations, voice problems, and language disorders. It is interesting that a disorder in the structure and function of seeing—like dyslexia—is not commonly considered a communicative disorder, except perhaps by some of those who have it. If one were to accept these four categories as exhaustive, then dyslexia (at least some aspects of it) would have to be included as a kind of language disorder; and, by analogy with certain aspects of central-pathway function related to hearing, that is very possibly where it belongs. The assessment of reading level and vocabulary range is a very important tool in the differential evaluation of communicative disorders, except for preschool-age children, and if these assessments are not generally made in speech and hearing clinics, they should be. In terms of prevalence, we should expect to find dyslexia quite commonly relatable to the general rubric "childhood aphasia"; it is frequently relatable to some forms of profound hearing impairment, particularly the kind currently labeled "dysacusis" which reflects disorders of auditory discrimination and recognition; it is rarely related to voice disorders. Perhaps more often than is commonly thought, dyslexia is clearly relatable to certain diagnostic categories used to describe aberrant speech. It may or may not be relatable, either directly or tangentially, to the various forms of adult aphasia.

Clearly all these possibilities cannot be explored in the time at our disposal. It may be fruitful to consider only a few in some detail. There are certain aspects of hearing, for instance, which may well be analogous to some of the particulars of seeing, and therefore of dyslexia. Fortunately, much of the auditory system in mammals is quite accessible for various kinds of anatomical, physiological, and behavioral studies; a vast amount of manpower and brainwork is currently being devoted to these studies, and the results are rewarding. Our neonates are equipped to respond to auditory stimulation; these are reflexive responses which develop in various refinements until, at about three to four months of age, an auditory orienting reflex is clearly discernible. Thereafter, the infant learns how to listen, discriminate, recognize, and remember various details of the auditory experience. Eventually, by about seven months of age, he hears well enough to be able to respond consistently to quite minimal sounds which interest him—Ewing and Ewing (1944). If, on the other hand, there are impairments at the level of the central pathways which affect recognition and temporal management of auditory stimuli, the stimuli may be unreinforced and profound sensory inhibition may occur—Mark and Hardy (1958). This was one of Pavlov's earliest "laws of conditioning." The net result may well be profound deafness despite a quite normal peripheral sense-organ. Aside from this sort of negative status, however, in ensuing developmental stages the infant is capable of many refinements of attention, inhibition, and learning so far as the day's events in sound are concerned.

It is clear that the normal auditory mechanism performs (or has) three basic functions: sensitivity, discrimination, and recognition— all relative to the three physical dimensions of sound: intensity, frequency, and phase. Deafness as a diagnostic term has classically been employed largely with problems of sensitivity. It is only fairly recently that psychoacoustic distortion (reflecting a dysfunction of sensitivity and discrimination) and dysacusis (reflecting a dysfunction of discrimination and recognition) have been clearly recognized as important attributes of profound hearing impairment. In terms of the nature of the auditory signal which reaches the cortex, there are major differences between hypoacusis and dysacusis. A similar distinction in terms of the detail of visual signals might be fruitful with regard to problems of dyslexia.

There are at least three other functions which involve the tracking of acoustic stimuli—related directly to hearing, dependent on hearing, but not *of* it in a behavioral sense: processing, pattern-making, and retention. These are evidently not functions of audition, but of what is done with the auditory input in terms of the total cerebral activity related to it. These are functions of the temporal management of the information contained in the auditory input. In this reference, processing means the ability to perceive rapidly successive bits of information; pattern-making means the capacity to relate this information in terms of significance to past and present behavior. In the total picture, both are subaspects of memory and recall, and are therefore associated with retention. Accordingly, fleeting attention, perseveration, and not-listening may all show behaviorally as inappropriate responses to sound without at all reflecting a lack of audition. Processing, pattern-making, and retention are not auditory functions, but, in this context, are dependent on the nature and extent of acoustic information that is coming through the system. Various models of cortical mechanisms for dealing with problems of temporal integration in serial-order have been suggested by Lashley (1951). Various distinctions relative to a sensory system and the information it processes are amenable to some measurement and analysis. These distinctions are important controlling concepts in the daily clinical tasks of differentiating among many kinds of hearing impairment, and between a disorder of hearing and a disorder of language comprehension and use. It seems reasonable that a similar analysis of vision, seeing, and the management of visual information in temporal terms might be useful in the study of dyslexia.

In assessing these attributes of sensory management, particularly in preschool-age children who are still in a prereading stage of development, we frequently find that a given child tested with non-verbal tasks has just as much difficulty in the serial-order temporal integration of visual information as he does with auditory. This is one reason why a careful definition of his visual language is important. A child who is only classically deaf, in terms of profound loss of auditory sensitivity, and who is not otherwise defective, is expected to show clear evidence of considerable facility in lipreading by the age of three. If he does not, the chances are very good that he has problems in the management of visual information.

Because of the size of our clinical load of children who do not evidently respond to sound or who do not communicate, we see much else than the classically deaf child. A large proportion of the preschool-age case load includes multiply impaired children, many of whom have no clear causal history. By and large, these children must be presumed to have a wide variety of developmental anomalies which do not lend themselves to classical descriptions. Some have a combination of hypoacusis, dysacusis, and profound problems in sensory temporal integration. Some of the motor palsied children have impaired hearing, language disorders, and dysarthrias. A few apparently have only motor language disabilities.

Most offer one aspect or another of emotional instability. The point that one is forced to consider with great care is that there are apt to be fundamental differences in both description and prediction between the so-called brain-injured child and the child with the kinds of central nervous system (CNS) peculiarities of management and attention that have been referred to. Some of the most subtle clinical problems in speech and hearing are those which do not show classical neurological symptoms, and which are therefore not subjects for classical neurological presumptions about brain injury. These children usually have CNS peculiarities; somewhere in the various reverberatory circuits of the brain, possibly involving several systems, there are inadequacies in the feedback circuitry. It seems entirely reasonable that this is what is involved in much of dyslexia—not just a twisting of orthographic details because of some lack of cerebral dominance, and not necessarily anything to do with a focal lack of tissue; but an inadequacy in the reinforcing mechanisms which make processing, pattern-formation, and retention possible and productive.

This idea seems clearly applicable to other kinds of communicative disorders, particularly two forms of deviant speech, infantile perseveration and cluttering. It has been the practice for many years to describe various articulatory disorders as organic or functional; those which are not central in cause are called dyslalias. One common form of dyslalia is infantile perseveration. The symptoms are common: a child, now six years old, continues to use the speech patterns which would be appropriate for a child thirty months old. These problems are often not easy to manage, for infantile speech perseveration does not happen by chance. A considerable number of these children are socially and emotionally immature, and many become slow or inadequate readers. It would be interesting, indeed, to document a relationship between a history of infantile perseveration of speech and dyslexia, with due attention paid to refined observations regarding auditory and visual memory. This sort of study cannot well be done in ordinary clinical follow-up work; the children are lost in the educative scheme of things, and the necessary relationships are not studied prospectively, but retrospectively.

A possible clue to this relationship, and to the general study of dyslexia, may be found in a quite straightforward clinical determination: the fact that many children with infantile speech perseveration do not naturally develop what might be called a critical auditory self-monitoring system. This is a communicative servomechanism that is important in the normal development of language and speech. It is usually apparent in the third to fourth year, and develops from normal habits of hearing and listening. The child learns to listen critically to his own speech in comparison with the speech he hears, and to match this with considerable fidelity in terms of idiom and dialectal detail. This observation was made by the ancient Greeks, who thought much of the importance of "ear training." Now called "auditory training," it is the basic remedial procedure employed by speech clinicians the world over when working with children with infantile speech perseveration. Of the children who cannot well learn this sort of critical auditory self-monitoring, it would be most interesting to know more precisely how many have problems in visual as well as in auditory processing and retention.

Speech deviation relative to this lack of monitoring is perhaps most obviously exemplified by the diagnostic entity called "cluttering." Some mild degree of cluttering is apparent in many forms of dyslalia; in its extreme form as a clinical entity, cluttering includes marked omissions and substitutions to a degree that approaches jargonic speech, and not uncommonly involves marked dysrhythmia. The subject knows what he wants to say; he intends to say it; but what comes out is phonetically garbled, usually with inappropriate stress-patterns. Some of these speech clutterers learn to read, and it may be that this achievement helps them to learn better phonic control of their speech. Many continue to offer various problems in academic learning. How many are genuine dyslexics remains to be determined. One might expect to find various common factors in processing and retention between cluttering and dyslexia.

In terms of a kind of hierarchical operational analysis of thought processes and problem solving, a very considerable amount of work has been done in the development of quite sensitive tests, particularly for the refined functions of temporal management under discussion.[1] It remains to study the possible relationships—causal, developmental, and behavioral—between hearing and speech disorders and dyslexia. It is too easy in clinical work in audiology and speech to pay attention only to the obvious symptoms, to measure hearing loss, to list the aberrant phonetic values, to work on the motor problems. Much more attention needs to be paid to the different, often quite subtle, anomalies of central sensory functions and their management in temporal integration relative to speech, hearing, language, and reading disorders.

By and large, and no doubt for various reasons, educators have considered that learning to read is specifically the business of education. Only quite recently have some educators come to realize that the inability to learn to read may have some causal basis that is relatable to the many factors which produce our atypical children. Apparently, as has happened in recent years with regard to most other forms of human communicative disorders, there needs to be a much closer relationship between clinical methods and findings and educative arts and skills—first, in an attempt to understand the nature of dyslexia in a given child; and then to learn how to do something productive about it.

[1] For instance, the work of Dr. Henry J. Mark and his associates at the Johns Hopkins Children's Diagnostic and Evaluation Center. Dr. Mark is preparing his findings for publication under the title, "A Theory of Thinking and the Logical Basis for Diagnosis, Classification, and Management of Behavioral Dysfunctions." See, Elementary thinking and the classification of behavior. Science, 135:75-87, 1962.

12

Dyslexia: Its Relationship to Language Acquisition and Concept Formation

JOSEPH M. WEPMAN

The present communication is directed toward an examination of the concept that the various factors involved in the maturation of the cognitive processes are all interrelated. Concept formation, oral language acquisition, and reading are viewed in this context as facets of the cognitive process, each contributing its share to the burgeoning development of thought in the early years of childhood. Each facet is seen as a steppingstone for the development of the next in a natural progression, when no impairment exists. The stream of development is not only seen as moving forward in a predictable chronological order, but also feeding back data as each matures, to enhance and stimulate the further development of its precursor. It is further held as a fundamental tenet that the mind of man is no empty transmitter of external environmental forces, but an active, dynamic process by which man interprets, integrates, and manipulates his environment to satisfy his own personal needs. The present paper concerns itself with the mechanisms by which it is thought that this "organ of the mind," to use Jackson's (Taylor [1931]) phrase, comes into being and develops.

While at first glance it may appear that some of the foregoing is somewhat tangential to the title, the opposite will be seen to be true. The importance of reading and the effect of reading impairment upon the total process of the development of cognition can most easily be demonstrated through the very interrelationships we seek to make explicit.

Dyslexia is used in the present paper to mean any or all degrees of reading impairment from nonreading to delays in the normal acquisition of reading of sufficient degree that the subject is considered a reading problem. With Robinson (1937) the author believes that dyslexia may be due to a number of factors and in many instances may have multiple causation. Of primary concern here will be those reading problems where it has been impossible to determine a specific etiology, and to provide a possible rationale for the cause of the defect.

The relationships we seek to clarify between concept formation, oral language acquisition and reading, or its impairment, are viewed in the context of the development of the neurological substrata which serve the increasing needs of the maturing child. Two relatively new neurological concepts serve as a background for the present construct. First, that the central nervous system differentiates both structurally and functionally during the early years of life. At the outset it functions as a reflex organism capable of simply transmitting stimuli along predetermined courses to stipulated motor expression (an almost one-to-one stimulus-response system). It then develops progressively through a series of levels permitting perceptual and finally conceptual function to ensue. At these higher levels signals are carried along specific input modalities, decoded and encoded, recognized, comprehended, retained in memory, associated with previously received stimuli and sensory images—in other words, they go through a process of integration before they become motor patterns along specific output modalities. The stimulus-response relationship at these higher levels is necessarily less direct and more tenuous in nature because of the multiplicity of events contributing to the response in the complexities of the integrative process. This interposition of a stage of integration which by its nature is not modality bound between input and output has its neurological confirmation in the work of Coghill (1929), Livingston, Haugen, and Brookhart (1954) and more recently in the studies of Penfield and Roberts (1959). A more complete exposition of the concept has been previously described in studies of the language of adult aphasic patients (Wepman, Jones, Bock, and Van Pelt [1960]).

The second major neurological tenet is that the pattern of development of the nervous system is largely genetic, namely, the order and the extent of neural differentiation, in terms of both the sensory modalities and the eventual level of conceptualization, is predetermined. The rate of development within the various modalities, however, is seen as being the product of external stimulation as well as internal striving to satisfy the needs of the total organism. This concept of the speed of maturation being determined by function, or, stated otherwise, the individual organism attempting new tasks and thereby forming new neural structure to accommodate the more complex organization required of it, follows the work of Coghill (1929), Edfeldt (1960), and others. Thus, some children who are in Charcot's (Freud [1953]) terms "audile," or of the ideational type where learning is easiest along the auditory modality, will bring to fruition those language functions dependent on audition earlier than will the children who are "visile." Oppositely, the "visile" child may be delayed in developing oral language, but does very much better when he approaches that part of the learning of language which calls for visual skill.

Viewing the factors under present discussion in the light of the foregoing, the interdependencies become evident. Concept formation in its prodromal state develops as the individual gains comprehension from his environment as his highest levels of neural structure develop. The concepts he can use are rudimentary and always related to very direct and immediate satisfaction of needs. If by genetic chance the child is visile, his stage of development into the use of oral language may be delayed. If, on the other hand, he is audile, he may develop oral language rapidly and accurately. Having, however, acquired this "alphabet of sounds," he can add to his concepts oral expression or the symbolic formulation of verbal forms based on the sequential patterning of his perceptual learning.

He can begin to speak. Through speech he can control and manip-
ulate his environment, the feedback from his oral effort can enhance
his concepts and his conceptual ability will increase with his spoken
vocabulary. While this may not be the sole source of his cognitive
development as some linguists hold (Whorf [1956]), the importance
of this language feedback seems evident, for it is through this
process that the usefulness of the concepts expressed become proven
and the likelihood of the future success in their use becomes
apparent.

The development of conceptual behavior and language is, in its
initial stages at least, confined to oral production based on auditory
perception. It is limited to temporal sequential processes since the
modality of perception is auditory and the stimuli evanescent.
Thought and language are usually concrete and stimulus-bound
since auditory learning depends for its stimulation on the immediate
presence of a producer.

It is not difficult to demonstrate the differential development of
children to this stage. Regarding the child's age for the acquisition
of its first words, note the excellent review by Darley and Winitz
(1961) of various studies that have been made. The age range
varies in these studies from a lower limit of four months (Terman
[1926]) to an upward limit of sixty months (Abt, Adler, and
Bartleme [1929]). While no attempt is made by the various authors
to stipulate a cause for the differences, the accepted close relationship between auditory development and language acquisition seems
adequate. Children develop oral language as they reach the stage
of auditory perception and concept formation sufficient to their
needs.

The differential development of audition and its consequences
relative to articulatory accuracy in speech have been reported in
the literature (Wepman [1960]; Wepman [1961]). Children with
slower developing auditory perception, especially auditory discrimination, are found generally to be (1) slower in beginning to talk
and (2) slower in acquiring speech accuracy. The fact that some
children do not develop adequate discrimination until they reach
the life age of eight, without one's needing to postulate either
pathology or mental deficiency, has been shown empirically. That

this is true has been known clinically for many years.

The next stage in the development of the child is when it acquires the capacity to learn vicariously, when it develops the neural integrative structure that permits the comprehension and concept-formation processes to mature through the substitutive learning of visual, orthographic symbols, when he learns to read. To acquire this ability he must follow one of two major pathways. Either his recognition and comprehension must be purely visual (this is the accepted belief of those who teach reading as a uniquely visual task) or he must associate his new visual learning with his previously acquired phonemic-phonetic learning. This latter viewpoint is strongly held by some authorities and researchers as the manner in which all children learn to read. Judd (1927), for example, stated that "oral language is the natural basis upon which the reading of beginners must be developed . . . recognition of printed words depends upon the analysis of visual sensory materials . . . these units must at first be made to coincide with their oral counterparts." Another accepted authority in the field of reading, Buswell (1947), held that "the reading process is basically a kind of perceptual learning in which visual symbols are perceived and related to already known auditory symbols of spoken language." More recently, Edfeldt (1960), reporting on his extensive studies in Sweden, stated that " . . . the support given to reading by speech is to begin with very great . . . Auditory and motor aids are a common characteristic in the process of learning to read."

To these and others, reading, the visual task, is dependent upon previous auditory learning. They represent the phonetic approach as against the earlier stated viewpoint of the visual sight recognition approach to the teaching of reading.

It is the argument of the present paper that both are right, but equally, both are wrong. Rather, it seems more precise in the light of the concept stated here to conclude that some children acquire reading solely as a visual skill, while others do so through a combined phonetic-phonemic-visual integration.

Dyslexia can be viewed in this context in a number of ways. One way would be that a reading disability would be closely related to a speech disability, if a child is poor in auditory development and is approached in reading by a phonetic method. This relationship is easily seen, since if, as Van Riper and Butler (1955) hold, the alphabet of letters and the alphabet of sounds are closely interrelated, then having an inadequate phonemic-phonetic pattern would lead to delayed development of speech and equally delayed acquisition of reading. Evidence for this is also to be found in the previously discussed studies of auditory discrimination (Wepman [1960]). In these studies with intelligence held constant, it was found that some 27 per cent of eighty children in the first grade showed inadequate auditory discrimination and reading scores significantly below the reading level of the children with adequate auditory discrimination. The developmental nature of the discriminatory learning is seen in that 19 per cent of children in the second grade showed a similar correlation. The studies of Goetzinger, Dirks, and Baer (1960) found very similar results using the same auditory discrimination tests (Wepman [1958]).

It needs only to be pointed out for the modality distinction that similar difficulties in reading are now being found in children with adequate auditory discrimination but inadequate development of prereading visual skills (Frostig, Lefever, and Whittlesey [1961]).

To return to one of the primary interrelations under discussion here, consider the extension of the maturation of cognition that comes with reading; and its opposite, the delayed development which may follow dyslexia. Concepts, as we have seen, are nurtured and develop through oral language, but are limited by the nature of the auditory modality upon which such language is based. As visual symbols became comprehensible and useful, however, no such limitations are necessary. The child as he acquires the ability to do his learning through the printed word also acquires the mechanism for greater abstraction. He is no longer bound to the temporal sequence of audition but develops the spatial sequences of vision—he learns that words substitute not only for the immediate here-and-now, but for the distant there-and-then, for the past and future as well as for the present to which he had been limited. It is easily seen how this new method of acquiring vocabulary materially extends and broadens the concept formation process. Now abstraction takes its most definitive form where the object to be abstracted is present only as a substitutive symbol, from the concrete present the individual matures to the abstracted past and future.

It is interesting at this point to postulate what this may mean to the child. We have been indebted to the insightful observations, now widely accepted, of Piaget (1955) for the concept that children change from an egocentric self to an ethnocentric, societal being at roughly the age of six. How coincidental it appears that this, too, is the age when most children learn to read—which is in another sense somewhat the same process, turning from the personal present to societal past and future. While Piaget concerned himself with the dynamic psychological factors leading to this change, with none of which I would disagree, yet the mechanism for this change has never been made explicit. It has just been said to occur when the personality needs of the child are such that he seeks external sources of satisfaction. The present concept, however, provides a more objective reason for the change. With the development of reading the potential for externalization becomes available; the wherewithal for turning outward becomes functional.

All of the foregoing relates to the normal child whose development follows the natural progression, whose ability to conceptualize is increased through the added impetus of reading. The dyslexic child, however, fails to develop the essential phase of cognitive maturation which permits the easy transition to ethnocentric adaptation. Off the cuff, since it has not yet been released for publication, it has been stated that in delinquency-prone areas the children who become delinquent are the nonreaders, while in the same population centers the children who learn to read are less likely to develop deviant antisocial behavior.

Neurologically, there may even be reason to point to the potential for decreased neural differentiation since if development here follows use, a lack of development would follow a lack of use.

Summary

This paper presents a concept of the potential for intense interrelationships between the factors underlying the development of cognition. The mechanism for the concept has been seen as the differential modality maturation in children thought to be due to inherent qualities largely genetically determined. The importance of the concept cannot be overstated. It implies that there are notable individual differences in children relative to the modality of learning and, following this, that reading in our schools should not be by a single approach, but rather one directed toward the capacities of the individual child. (Methods are now available and others being developed which permit the identification of the maximal learning modality of the child during his formative, preschool years.) It implies that a sizable number of dyslexic children are so, not because of any specific brain damage, personality problem, or immaturity, but rather because they have been improperly taught. It stresses the fact that reading is not a visual skill alone for all children, but for some may be the integration of many skills; and that dyslexia's effect upon the person can be seen as more than a disability in reading: it is also a vital factor in intellectual and psychological maturation. To quote Hermann (1959), "not the eyes but the brain learns to read."

13

Reading Difficulties as a Neurological Problem in Childhood

HEINZ F. R. PRECHTL

From the neurological point of view, we may divide reading disabilities into two groups: a first group with lesions in specific cerebral structures which deal with the function of reading, e.g., the brain areas 17, 18 and 19, which subserve a visual but non-language function, and area 39, which combines both visual and language functions; and a second group with nonspecific lesions of the central nervous system in which the performance of reading is impaired in general, more or less as a side effect. I would like to deal here with this second group.

In the literature, minor neurological abnormalities have been mentioned in children with developmental dyslexia. Rabinovitch and his co-workers (1954) described in some cases a delay in the ability to appreciate the double nature when face and hand were stimulated simultaneously. Frequently a confusion of left and right was found. And "observation of gait and the performance of motor acts such as dressing, opening and closing doors, and the handling of psychological test materials led to the definite impression of a nonspecific awkwardness and clumsiness in motor function." Similar observations have been described by other workers. Bakwin and Bakwin (1960) said about children with reading disabilities: "A considerable proportion of affected children are abnormally clumsy. Their movements are jerky, uncoordinated and bungling. . . . The condition is evident in early childhood, but becomes more prominent during the school years." Recently a more detailed neurological study has been published by Cohn (1961). He compared a group of 46 children having reading and writing difficulties with 130 randomly chosen children, who were in normal schoolroom classes and did not overtly show the awkwardness mentioned above. Striking differences between both groups were found in right-left orientation, in the evaluation of double simultaneous tactile stimuli, the knee-jerk reflexes, the Babinski sign, the motor coordination, the mechanics of speech and the EEG.

These studies offer some evidence that many of the children with reading difficulties suffer from "minimal brain damage." This view is supported by other studies which have shown a high incidence of pre- or paranatal complications in the history of children with reading problems (Eustis [1947]; Eames [1955], Kawi and Pasamanick [1958]), suggesting again the occurrence of abnormalities of the central nervous system.

Our own efforts were primarily directed toward the possibility of picking out a uniform neurological syndrome among the many heterogeneous groups of hyperkinetic children who had been referred to a neurologist, mainly because of poor school performance: Prechtl and Stemmer (1959; 1962). It was noticed, while EEGs were being taken, that very many of these children—aged seven to fourteen years—exhibited in varying degrees distinct chorealike twitchings of the extremities and of the head, which showed up on the EEG as muscle artifacts from the cervical and temporal muscles. In some cases these movements were so pronounced that they were at first thought to be of an infectious origin, in fact rheumatic chorea.

Starting from these accidental observations, we made a systematic investigation of a group of 50 children from nine to twelve years old who, apart from the presence of choreiform movements, were selected on the basis only of age. Children with other obvious neurological signs (e.g., those with cerebral palsy, microcephaly, etc.) or psychiatric symptoms (e.g., mental subnormality) were excluded. Besides an exhaustive case history, the investigation consisted of a thorough neurological examination, laboratory tests (blood, urine and sometimes cerebrospinal fluid), at least two EEGs and an EKG, serological tests for rheumatism and toxoplasmosis, and in some cases a pneumoencephalogram. In addition, electromyograms were taken from some children using both needle and skin electrodes.

We selected only those patients who showed choreiform movements, by which we mean slight jerky movements, occurring quite irregularly and arhythmically in different muscles. Their main characteristic is their sudden occurrence and short duration which distinguish them clearly from slow tonic athetoid movements. Electromyographic analysis makes this even plainer. There is a short phasic discharge, which normally is produced in the electromyogram only by tendon reflexes (e.g., from the quadriceps muscle in the knee jerk).

Not only do these choreiform discharges occur in contracted muscles, producing a small movement, but they can also be detected electromyographically in fully relaxed muscles where there is no visible movement. This observation shows why clinically the choreiform restlessness is the greater, the higher the general muscle tone; and why it clearly becomes less when the muscles are relaxed. One can understand choreiform activity being more clearly visible in "stress situations."

While the muscles of the tongue, face, neck, and trunk were involved in 100 per cent of the cases (this and other percentages refer to the 50 children whom we examined), in 18 per cent we found the choreiform movements in the distal muscles of the extremities but less clear than in the trunk and head. We called that which occurred in 82 per cent of our group, the "proximal form."

In 96 per cent of the children the eye muscles were also affected, causing disturbances of conjugate movement and difficulty in fixation and reading. In some cases we could correlate errors in word recognition with the occurrence of involuntary eye movements by recording an electrooculogram during reading. It seems at least sensible to suppose that this difficulty in fixation may lead to considerable functional disturbance.

The tendon reflexes were normal in only 18 per cent—the rest noticeably exaggerated. In 66 per cent clonic aftercontractions followed the knee-jerk reflex. Differences between right and left did not occur. Muscle tone was normal in 76 per cent, high in 14 per cent, and only 10 per cent could be said to show hypotonia. In testing for muscle tone by passive movements of the extremities and palpation of the muscles the choreiform twitches could be clearly felt. It was at times reminiscent of a cogwheel phenomenon but the resistance to passive movement was too irregular to cause any confusion.

A disturbance in coordination (finger-nose, and heel-knee tests) depended on the intensity of the choreiform twitches, but this was always due to dyskinesia and not to a true ataxia.

There were no gross disturbances in sensation, especially not in stereognosis, but most of the children had difficulties in left and right discrimination. Although there was only one boy who was left-handed, 58 per cent could be called ambilateral.

The Behavior of Children with Choreiform Movements

As I have already remarked above, these children were brought to the doctor not on account of any neurological condition, but because of behavior disorders at home and poor schoolwork. But the question arises whether there is a causal relationship between these neurological and behavioral phenomena or whether both are the effect of a common cause. To begin with, it is quite obvious that a child's psychic development may be disturbed by a motor disorder, in particular when the disorder affects the capacity for delicate movements of the eyes or hands. The afferent impulses, optical, postural and tactile, which are transmitted to the nervous system are rendered slightly false or inadequate by the motor dyskinesia, which affects the child's relationship with his environment or at least inhibits its normal development. This alone would suffice to explain the difficulties of our patients in reading and writing, and the frequency of disordered spatial perception and orientation. And in fact 90 per cent of the group of 50 children had more or less trouble in reading. In all of them the choreiform activity involved the eye muscles.

In another study, being carried out at the moment by Stemmer, additional evidence is accumulated that children with the choreiform syndrome are poor readers and show a significantly lower performance in their schoolwork than a control group. On the other hand, in a population study, Dr. Stemmer found a significantly different distribution of the choreiform syndrome in regular schools and special schools for children with learning difficulties.

The majority of our 50 subjects' parents declared that, even at an early age, their children had displayed particularly unrestrained, wild behavior, clumsiness, inability to concentrate on any plaything for long, and very labile moods fluctuating between timidity and outbursts of aggression. The obtrusive symptoms clearly distinguished these children from their siblings. Therefore, it seems very improbable that harmful environments or other psychological or socioeconomic factors were the cause of the behavior disorders. When the children were sent to school their behavior became increasingly intolerable. At school those very abilities are required which children with a choreiform syndrome do not possess: sitting still or concentrating on a subject for long periods, differentiated functions of fine motor control in writing and reading and, lastly, adjustment of emotional life to a new community—often very trying even for healthy children. The child's understandable failure produces reactions, which in their turn lead to new burdens such as impositions, constant admonishments from teachers, and so on. Such children are caught in a vicious circle, and become progressively more and more neurotic either to the point of a breakdown or, as sometimes happens, until an understanding adult demands help for them.

However, in most cases the behavioral abnormalities already mentioned contrast with a rapid functional development and a basically lively intelligence. These children stand and walk in time

and are alert and active, and at first promise much more than they
are able to fulfill later—facts which disguise the existence of cerebral injury and cause parents to be disappointed at their children's
subsequent failures.

In short: the laboratory findings were that the patients showed
no abnormalities. The EEG showed spikes in tracings typical of epileptic discharges in seven cases; in the other 43 cases the EEG was
normal or more labile in response to hyperventilation or flicker
stimulation than the control group. But, in all EEGs, short muscle
artifacts appeared from the leads over the temporal and neck
muscles and did not do so in the control group.

Very striking were the case histories according to the reports
given by the parents. In 50 per cent the course of pregnancy was
complicated by toxemia, severe bleedings, etc. In 46 per cent of
the children neonatal disturbances occurred (26 per cent had been
treated for severe asphyxia; 14 per cent had difficulties in sucking
and had a low body temperature; in 8 per cent the delivery was
premature).

In 60 per cent of our patients we found a history of illness in their
postnatal development: 28 per cent had episodes of cyanosis in
early life, complicated pneumonia or pertussis infections; 12 per
cent had frequent epileptic attacks. In no less than 38 per cent
there was a history of accidents with concussion. The last point
demonstrates that these children are accident-prone, as has been
demonstrated in another study going on in our hospital (Dr.
Wouters), showing that about 80 per cent of the children who had
one or even more accidents in their history are choreatic. Only
19 per cent of another, nonchoreatic group had accidents.

Summing up these findings we may say: Out of a group of children with learning problems, a distinct neurological syndrome occurs in a number of them, suggesting the presence of minimal brain
damage. These findings contrast with other reports in which the
hereditary character of reading disability is stressed (Hallgren
[1950]; and others). Hermann and Norrie (1958) suggested that
specific dyslexia (word blindness) is a congenital type of Gerstmann's syndrome. It is evident, however, that our children with
the choreiform syndrome are a different group. My suggestion is

that some of the children with reading difficulties have these problems because they cannot fixate longer and have a quite serious instability of concentration caused by the choreiform activity. These defects in their neural function may also lead to a lag in the development of cerebral dominance and to a delay in the development of complex functions as, for instance, reading. However, we found a few children without learning difficulties although they suffered from a severe form of the choreiform syndrome; all of them have an IQ higher than 130 and it seems that they can compensate for their troubles.

These remarks are still hypothetical and very incomplete. We hope to continue our research and come to a better understanding of the influence of the dysfunctions of the nervous system on dyslexia.

Glossary

agnosia: inability to interpret sensory impression; loss of ability to recognize and identify familiar objects through a particular sense organ. In *visual* or *optic agnosia*, there is loss of ability to recognize objects in the visual field, due to lesions in the cerebral cortex, although the person is not blind in the ordinary sense of not seeing.

anoxia: deficiency or lack of oxygen. It may occur in the newborn in the transition from maternal supply of oxygenated cord blood to independent breathing. The brain cells are particularly vulnerable to continued anoxia.

aphasia: defect or loss of the power of expression by speech, writing, or signs, or of comprehending spoken or written language, due to injury or disease of the brain centers.

apraxia: loss of ability to perform purposeful movements, in the absence of paralysis or sensory disturbance; caused by lesions in the cerebral cortex.

astereognosis: a form of agnosia in which there is a loss of power to recognize objects or to appreciate their form by touching or feeling them.

ataxia: marked incoordination in movements of the voluntary musculature.

athetosis: a derangement of muscular movement, resulting principally from brain lesion, marked by slow, recurring, weaving movements of arms and legs, and by facial grimaces.

195

Babinski sign: the extensor-plantar response. There is extension of the toes instead of flexion on stimulating the sole of the foot. It is an aid to neurological diagnosis.

body image: the picture or mental representation one has of one's own body at rest or in motion at any moment. It is derived from internal sensations, postural changes, contact with outside objects and people, emotional experiences and fantasies. *Body image* is also a synonym of *body concept,* meaning one's evaluation of one's own body, with special attention on how one thinks or fantasies that it looks to others.

body schema: the over-all pattern of one's direct or sensory awareness of one's own body; the characteristic way in which a person is aware of his own body. The *body image* is an actual experience; the *body schema* is a pattern, an acquired structure that codetermines the body image in a given situation.

callosal: pertaining to the *corpus callosum.*

chorea: a neurological disorder characterized by jerky involuntary movements, or spasms of short duration, involving a considerable set of muscles.

choreiform: movements similar to those of chorea.

cluttering: bursting, "nervous" speech marked by frequent omissions and substitutions of sounds.

CNS: central nervous system.

cogwheel phenomenon: a sign of neurological disease of the brain. The arm is resistant to movement except in jerky motion, as of a cogwheel. It is seen most commonly in the neurological examination of adults with Parkinsonism.

corpus callosum: if the two hemispheres of the cerebral cortex were the meat of a walnut, then the corpus callosum would be the outermost covering of the topside of the core that joins the two halves together.

cyanosis: blueness of the skin, due to insufficient oxygen in the blood, as a result of poor circulation or, especially in the newborn, delayed or insufficient breathing.

dysacusis: hearing impairment which involves distortion of loudness or pitch, or both, rather than loss in sensitivity.

dysarthria: an articulatory disorder reflecting CNS dysfunction of the motor musculature of speech. Cf. dyslalia.

dyskinesia: impairment of the power of voluntary movement, resulting in fragmentary or incomplete movements, poorly coordinated.

dyslalia: defective articulation caused by factors other than CNS dysfunction. Cf. dysarthria.

dysrhythmia: abnormal speech fluency, usually characterized by defective stress, breath control, and intonation.

EEG: electroencephalogram, or brainwave tracing.

EKG: electrocardiogram, a graphic tracing of the changes in electric potential of heart muscle produced by contractions of the heart.

electromyogram: a graphic tracing which records the changes of electric potential in a contracting muscle.

electro oculogram: an electrographic tracing from eye muscles.

feedback: in an organism, the sensory report of the somatic result of behavior, e.g., the kinesthetic report that indicates the speed and extent of a movement; or the pain that follows the touching of a hot object. Cf. servomechanism.

Gestalt: a form, a configuration, or a totality that has, as a unified whole, properties which cannot be derived by summation from the parts and their relationships. Plural: Gestalts or Gestalten.

global: in psychology and behavior theory, total; taken as a whole without attempt to distinguish separate parts or functions, e.g., a global response to brain stimulation.

gnosia: the faculty of perceiving and knowing.

gnosic: pertaining to gnosia.

hemianopia: blindness in one half of the field of vision in one or both eyes.

hemianopia, homonymous: one which affects the nasal half of one eye and the contrary, i.e. temporal half of the other. In other words, either the left half of each retina is affected, or the right half. The optic tracts from the left side of each retina go to the left hemisphere of the brain, and from the right side of each retina to the right hemisphere. Thus, half of the vision from each eye, the temporal half, is represented in the *same* side of the brain and is not crossed as is the representation of the arms and legs. The nasal half of the vision from each eye is represented in the opposite brain hemisphere. See Fig. 4, p. 123; and p. 129.

hypoacusis: hearing impairment which involves loss in sensitivity; it may be conductive or sensori-neural, or mixed.

idiopathic: self-originated; of unknown origin.

information theory: an interdisciplinary study, of which communications theory is the technology, dealing with the transmission of messages or signals, or the communication of information. It draws upon physics, engineering, cybernetics, linguistics, psychology, and sociology.

interoceptor: a sense organ or receptor inside the body, in contrast with an exteroceptor at or near the surface. Adj., interoceptive.

ipsilateral: homolateral; occurring on the same side, e.g., the rare association of left-handedness and ipsilateral brain dominance for speech.

lobes of the brain: diagram of the left hemisphere of the cerebral cortex:

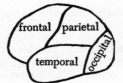

Lorge Magazine Count: a tabulation of the frequencies of occurrence of words in 4.59 million words of text from the five American magazines with the highest circulation in the period 1929-1938. It is generally accepted as the best source for estimating average word frequencies in English. Reference: E. L. Thorndike and I. Lorge, The Teacher's Word Book of 30,000 Words. New York, Teachers College, Columbia University, 1944.

macula: the macula lutea, an oval depression at the center of the retina of the eye which is the point of clearest vision.

muscle artifact: an irregularity in an EEG tracing produced as the electrical accompaniment of a movement of a voluntary muscle.

null hypothesis: in a typical experimental design, the hypothesis is that two variables show a greater-than-chance difference. The null hypothesis is that there is no difference greater than could be expected by chance; this is tested by statistical evaluation of obtained differences. If the null hypothesis can be proved false, its contradictory is thereby proved true.

paranatal: connected with or occurring during the birth process.

perserveration of infantile speech: the prolongation of articulatory habits appropriate, say, to the age period extending from 30 months to 60 or 70 months.

pneumoencephalogram: an electroencephalogram taken after the injection of air or gas into the ventricular spaces of the brain.

proprioceptor: a receptor or sense organ sensitive to the position and movement of the body and its members; they are found in the vestibule of the inner ear, the nearby semicircular canals, and in the muscles, tendons, and joints. Adj., proprioceptive.

self-monitoring: critical control of the phonetic details of speech by imitation through hearing and listening.

servomechanism: a control system (e.g., thermostat) for maintaining the operation of another system (e.g., furnace) at prescribed rates and strengths. The servomechanism receives a signal showing the amount of energy (the input) supplied to the operation system and a feedback signal showing the rate, strength, and/or direction of the operation (the output). The response of the "servo" to these signals regulates the input so that a prescribed output is maintained.

Snellen chart: the test types assembled by Snellen for ocular testing and very widely used.

splenium: the rear part of the corpus callosum.

stereognosis: perception of objects or forms by touch.

strephosymbolia: etymologically means "twisted symbols." The term was first used by Orton to denote difficulty in learning to read without evidence of other, gross mental defect. It also denotes a condition in which objects seem reversed, as in a mirror.

tachistoscope: an apparatus in psychology used for exposing colors, figures or other visual stimuli for fractions of a second.

teleoreceptor: a sensory nerve ending, as in the eyes, ears and nose, which is stimulated by a distant stimulus.

toxemia of pregnancy: a kind of blood poisoning associated with abnormal changes of body chemistry during pregnancy and producing a variety of symptoms including nausea, vomiting, shortness of breath, albumin in the urine and convulsions.

type-token ratio: in linguistics, a word is counted as a type for only one of its occurrences in a given utterance, that is, the first time it appears and not on repetitions; whereas each word and all its repetitions are counted as tokens. Thus: "The man saw the man," contains 3 types and 5 tokens, with a ratio of 3:5.

Wada sodium amytal test: a method introduced by Wada in 1949 for determining cerebral dominance. A one-sided intracarotid injection of sodium amytal is carried in the carotid artery directly to the same side of the brain. If it is the side of the dominant hemisphere, there will rapidly be disturbance of speech and a feeling of depression. On the nondominant side, there will be *no* language disturbance, and euphoria instead of depression. In both instances, EEG and other neurological signs are *unilateral*.

word-attack skills: a pedagogical term that refers to a child's ability to analyze unfamiliar words by syllables and phonic elements and so arrive at their pronunciation and possibly recognize their meaning.

Consolidated Bibliography

Abbott, C. 1882.   The intelligence of batrachians. Science, 3:66-67.

Abt, I. A., Adler, H. A., and Bartleme, P. 1929.   The relationship between the onset of speech and intelligence. Journal of the American Medical Association, 93:1351-1355.

Akelaitis, A. J. 1941.   Studies on the corpus callosum. II: The higher visual functions in each homonymous field following complete section of the corpus callosum. Archives of Neurology and Psychiatry, 45:788-796.

Akelaitis, A. J. 1943.   Studies on the corpus callosum. VII: Study of language functions (tactile and visual lexia and graphia) unilaterally following section of the corpus callosum. Journal of Neuropathology and Neurology, 2:226-262.

Akelaitis, A. J. 1944.   A study of gnosis, praxia and language following section of the corpus callosum and anterior commissure. Journal of Neurosurgery, 1:94-102.

Alajouanine, T., Lhermitte, F., and de Ribaucourt-Ducarne, B. 1960.   Les alexies agnosiques et aphasiques. In Les Grandes Activités du Lobe Occipital. Paris: Masson. P. 235.

Altus, G. T. 1956.   A WISC profile for retarded readers. Journal of Consulting Psychology, 20:155-156.

American Psychological Association. Committee on Test Standards. 1954. Technical recommendations for psychological tests and diagnostic techniques. Psychological Bulletin, 51, No. 2, Part 2.

Arthur, G. 1940.   Therapy with retarded readers. Journal of Consulting Psychology, 4:173-176.

Axline, V. M. 1947. Non-directive therapy for poor readers. Journal of Consulting Psychology, 11:61-69.

Bachmann, F. 1927. Über kongenitale Wortblindheit (Angeborene Leseschwäche). Abhandlungen aus der Neurologie, Psychiatrie, Psychologie und ihren Grenzgebieten, 40:1-72.

Bakwin, H. 1950. Psychiatric aspects of pediatrics: lateral dominance, right- and left-handedness. Journal of Pediatrics, 36:385-391.

Bakwin, H., and Bakwin, R. M. 1960. *Clinical Management of Behavior Disorders in Children.* (2nd edition). Philadelphia-London: W. B. Saunders Co.

Barger, W. C., Lavin, R., and Speight, F. S. 1957. Constitutional aspects in psychiatry of poor readers. Diseases of the Nervous System, 18:289-294.

Bastian, H. C. 1898. *A Treatise on Aphasia and Other Speech Defects.* London: H. K. Lewis.

Baxter, D. W., and Bailey, A. A. 1961. Primary reading epilepsy. Neurology, 11:445-449.

Bender, L. 1954. *A Dynamic Psychopathology of Childhood.* Springfield, Ill.: Charles C. Thomas.

Bender, L. 1956a. *Psychopathology of Children with Organic Brain Disorders.* Springfield, Ill.: Charles C. Thomas.

Bender, L. 1956b. Research studies from Bellevue Hospital on specific reading disabilities: résumé. Bulletin of the Orton Society, 6:1-3.

Bender, L. 1957. Specific reading disability as a maturational lag. Bulletin of the Orton Society, 7:9-18.

Benton, A. L. 1958. Significance of systematic reversal in right-left discrimination. Acta Psychiatrica et Neurologica Scandinavica, 33:129-137.

Benton, A. L. 1959. *Right-Left Discrimination and Finger Localization: Development and Pathology.* New York: Paul C. Hoeber.

Benton, A. L., and Kemble, J. D. 1960. Right-left orientation and reading disability. Psychiatry and Neurology, 139:49-60.

Bickford, R. G., Whelan, J. L., Klass, D. W., and Corbin, K. B. 1956. Reading epilepsy: clinical and electroencephalographic studies of a new syndrome. Transactions of the American Neurological Association, 81st Meeting, 100-102.

Bills, R. E. 1950. Non-directive play therapy with retarded readers. Journal of Consulting Psychology, 14:140-149.

Bingley, T. 1958. Mental symptoms in temporal lobe epilepsy and temporal lobe gliomas. Acta Psychiatrica et Neurologica Scandinavica, 33, Supp. 120.

Birch, H. G., and Bortner, M. 1960. Perceptual and perceptual-motor dissociation in brain-damaged patients. Journal of Nervous and Mental Disease, 130:49-53.

Birch, H. G., and Bortner, M. 1962. Perceptual and perceptual-motor dissociation in cerebral palsied children. Journal of Nervous and Mental Disease. In press.

Bouillaud, J. 1864-1865.   Discussion du rapport de Lélut. Bulletin de l'Académie de Médecine, Paris. Vol. 30.

Brain, W. R. 1945.   Speech and handedness. Lancet, 2:837-842.

Bramwell, B. 1899.   On "crossed aphasia" and the factors which go to determine whether the "leading" or "driving" speech centres shall be located in the left or in the right hemisphere of the brain, with notes on a case of "crossed" aphasia (aphasia with right-sided hemiplegia in a left-handed man). Lancet, 1:1473-1479.

Broadbent, W. H. 1872.   On the cerebral mechanism of speech and thought. Medico-Chirurgical Transactions, 55:145-194.

Broca, P. 1865.   Sur la faculté du langage articulé. Bulletin de la Société d'Anthropologie, 6:493-494.

Bronner, A. F. 1917.   *The Psychology of Special Abilities and Disabilities.* Boston: Little, Brown.

Buros, O. K. (ed.) 1953.   *The Fourth Mental Measurements Yearbook.* Highland Park, N. J.: Gryphon Press.

Buros, O. K. (ed.) 1959.   *The Fifth Mental Measurements Yearbook.* Highland Park, N. J.: Gryphon Press.

Burt, C. 1950.   *The Backward Child.* (3rd edition). London: University of London Press.

Buswell, G. T. 1947.   The sub-vocalization factor in the improvement of reading. Elementary School Journal, 48:190-196.

California Test Bureau. 1957.   *Technical Report on the California Achievement Tests.* (1957 edition.) Los Angeles.

Carmichael, E. A. 1954.   Hemispherectomy and the localization of function. In Lectures on the Scientific Basis of Medicine, 3:93-103.

Carnvale, E. 1961.   The etiology of reading disability. Laboratory report no. 2. Community Projects Section, Mental Health Study Center. Mimeographed manuscript.

Casey, T., and Ettlinger, G. 1960.   The occasional "independence" of dyslexia and dysgraphia from dysphasia. Journal of Neurology, Neurosurgery and Psychiatry, 23:228-236.

Cattell, J. M.   Über die Zeit der Erkennung und Benennung von Schriftzeichen, Bildern und Farben. Philosophische Studien (Wundt), 1885, 2:635-649.

Clemmens, R. L. 1961.   Minimal brain damage in children, an interdisciplinary problem: medical, para-medical and educational. Children: An Interdisciplinary Journal for the Professions Serving Children, 8:179-183.

Coghill, G. E. 1929.   *Anatomy and the Problem of Behavior.* Cambridge: Cambridge University Press.

Cohn, R. 1961a.   Delayed acquisition of reading and writing abilities in children: a neurological study. Archives of Neurology, 4:153-164.

Cohn, R. 1961b.   Dyscalculia. Archives of Neurology, 4:301-307.

Conrad, K. 1949.   Über aphasische Sprachstörungen bei hirnverletzten Linkshänder. Nervenarzt, 20:148-154.

Critchley, M. 1953.   *The Parietal Lobes*. Baltimore: Williams & Wilkins.

Cronbach, L. J., and Meehl, P. E. 1955.   Construct validity in psychological tests. Psychological Bulletin, 52:281-302.

Darley, F. L., and Winitz, H. 1961.   Age of first word. Journal of Speech and Hearing Disorders, 26:272-290.

Dejerine, J. 1892.   Contribution a l'étude anatamo-pathologique et clinique des différentes variétés de cécité verbale. Mémoires de la Société de Biologie, 4:61.

Delacato, C. H. 1959.   *The Treatment and Prevention of Reading Problems*. Springfield, Ill.: Charles C. Thomas.

Drew, A. L. 1956.   A neurological appraisal of familial congenital word-blindness. Brain, 79:440-460.

Eames, T. H. 1955.   The relationship of birth weight, the speeds of object and word perception, and visual acuity. Journal of Pediatrics, 47:603-606.

Ebel, R. L. 1961.   Must all tests be valid? American Psychologist, 16:640-647.

Edfeldt, A. W. 1960.   *Silent Speech and Silent Reading*. Chicago: University of Chicago Press.

Espir, M., and Russell, W. R. 1961.   *Traumatic Aphasia*. London: Oxford University Press. In Press.

Ettlinger, G., and Jackson, C. V. 1955.   Organic factors in developmental dyslexia. Proceedings of the Royal Society of Medicine, 48:998-1000.

Ettlinger, G., Jackson, C. V., and Zangwill, O. L. 1955.   Dysphasia following right temporal lobectomy in a right-handed man. Journal of Neurology, Neurosurgery and Psychiatry, 18:214-217.

Ettlinger, G., Jackson, C. V., and Zangwill, O. L. 1956.   Cerebral dominance in sinistrals. Brain, 79:569-588.

Ettlinger, G., Warrington, E., and Zangwill, O. L. 1957.   A further study of visual-spatial agnosia. Brain, 80:335-361.

Eustis, R. S. 1947.   The primary etiology of the specific language disabilities. Journal of Pediatrics, 31:448-455.

Ewing, I. R., and Ewing, A. W. G. 1944.   Ascertainment of deafness in infancy and early childhood. Journal of Laryngology and Otology, 59:309-333.

Ferguson-Smith, M. A. 1961.   Chromosomes and human disease. In *Progress in Medical Genetics*. New York: Grune & Stratton. Pp. 292-334.

Fernald, G. M. 1943.   *Remedial Techniques in Basic School Subjects*. New York: McGraw-Hill Book Co.

Filbin, R. L. 1957.   Prescription for the Johnny who can't read. Elementary English, 34:559-561.

Fildes, L. G. 1921. A psychological inquiry into the nature of the condition known as congenital word-blindness. Brain, 44:286-307.

Foix, C., and Hillemand, P. 1925. Rôle vraisemblable du splénium dans la pathogénie de l'alexie pure par lésion de la cérébrale postérieure. Bulletins et Mémoires de la Société Médicale des Hospitaux de Paris, 49:393.

Freud, S. 1953. *On Aphasia*. New York: International Universities Press.

Frostig, M. 1961. *Developmental Test of Visual Perception*. Published by the author: 7257 Melrose Ave., Los Angeles 46, Cal.

Frostig, M., Lefever, D. W., and Whittlesey, J. 1961. A developmental test of visual perception. Perceptual and Motor Skills, 12:383-394.

Galifret-Granjon, N. 1952. Le problème de l'organisation spatiale dans les dyslexies d'évolution. In *L'Apprentissage de la Lecture et ses Troubles*, Pp. 445-479. Paris: Presses Universelles France.

Galifret-Granjon, N., and Ajuriaguerra, J. de. 1951. Trouble de l'apprentissage de la lecture et dominance latérale. Encéphale, 3:385-398.

Gallagher, J. 1960. Specific language disability: dyslexia. Bulletin of the Orton Society, 10:5-10.

Gates, A. I. 1922. *The Psychology of Reading and Spelling with Special Reference to Disability*. Teachers College Contributions to Education, No. 129. Teachers College, Columbia University.

Gerstmann, J. 1924. Fingeragnosie. Eine umschriebene Störung der Orientierung am eigenen Körpor. Wiener klinische Wochenschrift, 37:1010-1012.

Gerstmann, J. 1940. Syndrome of finger agnosia, disorientation for right and left, agraphia and acalculia. Archives of Neurology and Psychiatry, 44:398-408.

Gerstmann, J. 1958. Psychological and phenomenological aspects of disorders of the body image. Journal of Nervous and Mental Disease, 126:499-512.

Geschwind, N. 1961. Quantitative studies of aphasic language. Paper read at the 7th International Congress of Neurology, Rome.

Geschwind, N., and Kaplan, E. 1962. A human cerebral deconnection syndrome: a preliminary report. Neurology. In press.

Getman, G. N. 1958. *How To Develop Your Child's Intelligence*. Published by the author: Luverne, Minn.

Gillingham, A. 1956. Part one, the prevention of scholastic failure due to specific language disability. Bulletin of the Orton Society, 6:26-31.

Gillingham, A., and Stillman, B. U. 1956. *Remedial Training for Children with Specific Disability in Reading, Spelling, and Penmanship*. (5th edition.) Distributed by Anna Gillingham, 25 Parkview Avenue, Bronxville, New York.

Goetzinger, C. P., Dirks, D. D., and Baer, C. J. 1960. Auditory discrimination and visual perception in good and poor readers. Annals of Otology, Rhinology and Laryngology, 69:121-136.

Goins, J. T. 1958. *Visual Perceptual Abilities and Early Reading Progress.*
Supplementary Educational Monographs, No. 87. Chicago: University of
Chicago Press.

Goldfarb, N. 1960. *An Introduction to Longitudinal Statistical Analysis.*
Glencoe, Ill.: Free Press.

Goodglass, H., and Quadfasel, F. A. 1954. Language laterality in left-
handed aphasics. Brain, 77:521-548.

Hallgren, B. 1950. Specific dyslexia ("congenital word-blindness"): a clinical and genetic study. Acta Psychiatrica et Neurologica Scandinavica,
Supp. 65.

Hambright, H. 1956. Part two, the prevention of scholastic failure due to
specific language disability. Bulletin of the Orton Society, 6:32-36.

Harmon, D. B. 1958. *Notes on a Dynamic Theory of Vision: A Study and
Discussion Outline.* Published by the author: Austin, Tex.

Harris, A. J. 1957. Lateral dominance, directional confusion and reading
disability. Journal of Psychology, 44:283-294.

Harris, A. J., and Roswell, F. G. 1953. Clinical diagnosis of reading disability. Journal of Psychology, 36:323-340.

Hebb, D. O. 1949. *The Organization of Behavior.* New York: John Wiley
& Sons.

Hécaen, H., Ajuriaguerra, J. de, and David, M. 1952. Les déficits fonction-
nels après lobectomie occipitale. Monatsschrift für Psychiatrie und
Neurologie, 123:239-291.

Hécaen, H., Ajuriaguerra, J. de, and Massonnet, J. 1951. Les troubles visuo-
constructifs par lésion pariéto-occipitale droite: rôle des perturbations
vestibulaires. L'Encéphale, 40:122-179.

Hécaen, H., and Piercy, M. F. 1956. Paroxysmal dysphasia and the problem
of cerebral dominance. Journal of Neurology, Neurosurgery and Psychiatry, 19:104-201.

Held, R. 1961. Exposure-history as a factor in maintaining stability of perception and coordination. Journal of Nervous and Mental Disease, 132:
26-32.

Held, R., and Bossom, J. 1961. Neonatal deprivation and adult rearrangement: complementary techniques for analyzing plastic sensory-motor co-
ordinations. Journal of Comparative and Physiological Psychology, 54:
33-37.

Hermann, K. 1956. Congenital word blindness. Acta Psychiatrica et Neurologica Scandinavica, Supp. 108:117-184.

Hermann, K. 1959. *Reading Disability: A Medical Study of Word-Blindness
and Related Handicaps.* Springfield, Ill.: Charles C. Thomas.

Hermann, K., and Norrie, E. 1958. Is congenital word-blindness a hereditary
type of Gerstmann's syndrome? Monatscchrift für Psychiatrie und Neurologie, 136:59-73.

Hilman, H. H. 1956. The effect of laterality on reading disability. Durham
Research Review, 7:86-96.

Hinshelwood, J. 1917. *Congenital Word-Blindness.* London: H. K. Lewis.

Hirsch, K. de. 1957. Tests designed to discover potential reading difficulties at the six-year-old level. American Journal of Orthopsychiatry, 27:566-576.

Hoff, H. 1961. Die Lokalisation der Aphasie. Paper read at the 7th International Congress of Neurology, Rome.

Holmes, G. 1950. Pure word blindness. Folia Psychiatrica Neurologica et Neurochirugica Neerlandics, 53:279.

Howes, D. H. 1961. Statistical properties of aphasic language. Paper read at the 7th International Congress of Neurology, Rome.

Howes, D. H. 1962. The form of the word-frequency effect. Psychologic Review. In press.

Howes, D. H., and Solomon, R. L. 1951. Visual duration threshold as a function of word-probability. Journal of Experimental Psychology, 41:401-410.

Humphrey, M. E., and Zangwill, O. L. 1952. Dysphasia in left-handed patients with unilateral brain lesions. Journal of Neurology, Neurosurgery and Psychiatry, 15:184-193.

Ingram, T. T. S. 1959. Specific developmental disorders of speech in childhood. Brain, 82:450-467.

Ingram, T. T. S. 1960. Paediatric aspects of specific developmental dysphasia, dyslexia and dysgraphia. Cerebral Palsy Bulletin, 2:254-277.

Ingram, T. T. S., and Reid, J. F. 1956. Developmental aphasia observed in a department of child psychiatry. Archives of Disease in Childhood, 31:161-172.

Jackson, J. H. 1868. Defect of intellectual expression (aphasia) with left hemiplegia. Lancet, 1:457-457.

Jackson, J. H. 1869. Abstract of Goulstonian Lectures on certain points on the study and classification of diseases of the nervous system. Lancet, 1:344; reprinted in Brain, 1915, 38:72-74.

Jackon, J. H. 1880. On aphasia, with left hemiplegia. Lancet, 1:637-638.

Johnson, M. 1961. Reading problems: diagnosis and treatment—A summary. Mimeographed manuscript. Temple University, Philadelphia.

Joss, L. W., Leiman, C. J., and Schiffman, G. B. 1961. An investigation of the value of remedial reading with psychotherapy in a public school system. Mimeographed manuscript. Board of Education, Baltimore County.

Jost, A. 1954. Hormonal factors in the development of the fetus. Cold Spring Harbor Symposia on Quantitative Biology, 19:167-181.

Judd, C. H. 1927. Reduction of articulation. American Journal of Psychology, 39:313-322.

Kallos, G. L., Grabow, J. M., and Guarino, E. A. 1961. The WISC profile of disabled readers. Personnel and Guidance Journal, Feb.: 476-478.

Kappel, S., and Bates, N. 1961. Epidemiology as a research method. Laboratory report no. 3, Community Progress Section, Mental Health Study Center. Mimeographed manuscript.

Karwoski, T. F., Gramlich, F. W., and Arnott, P. 1944.   Psychological studies in semantics. I: Free association reactions to words, drawings and objects. Journal of Social Psychology, 20:233-247.

Kawi, A. A., and Pasamanick, B. 1958.   Association of factors of pregnancy with reading disorders in childhood. Journal of the American Medical Association, 166:1420-1423.

Kawi, A. A., and Pasamanick, B. 1959.   Prenatal and paranatal factors in the development of childhood reading disorders. Monographs of the Society for Research in Child Development. Vol. 24, No. 4.

Kennard, M. A., Rabinovitch, R. D., and Wexler, D. 1952.   The abnormal electroencephalogram as related to reading disability in children with disorders of behavior. Canadian Medical Association Journal, 67:330-333.

Kohler, I. 1951.   Über Aufbau und Wandlungen der Wahrnehmungswelt. Vienna: Rudolph M. Rohrer.

Kuromaru, S., and Okada, S. 1961.   On developmental dyslexia in Japan. Paper read at the 7th International Congress of Neurology, Rome.

Lachmann, F. M. 1960.   Perceptual-motor development in children retarded in reading ability. Journal of Consulting Psychology, 24:427-431.

Langman, M. P. 1960.   The reading process: a descriptive, interdisciplinary approach. Genetic Psychology Monographs, 62:3-40.

Lashley, K. S. 1929.   *Brain Mechanisms and Intelligence.* Chicago: University of Chicago Press.

Lashley, K. S. 1951.   The problem of serial order in behavior. In *Cerebral Mechanisms in Behavior. The Hixon Symposium* (L. A. Jeffress, ed.). New York: John Wiley & Sons. Pp. 112-135.

Lecky, P. 1945.   *Self-Consistency: A Theory of Personality.* New York: Island Press.

Lewis, H. W. Jr. 1961.   A study of reading levels: standardized tests and informal tests. Mimeographed manuscript. The Reading Clinic, Public Schools of the District of Columbia.

Liepmann, H. 1908.   *Drei Aufsätze aus dem Apraxiegebiet.* Berlin: Karger.

Livingston, W. K., Haugen, F. P., and Brookhart, J. M. 1954.   Functional organization of the central nervous system. Neurology, 4:485-496.

Luria, A. R. 1947.   *Traumatic Aphasia: Its Syndromes, Pschopathology and Treatment.* An unpublished English translation is available by courtesy of the author; the original is published in Moscow by the Academy of Medical Sciences.

Lyman, R. S., Kwan, S. T., and Chao, W. H. 1938.   Left occipito-parietal brain tumor. With observations on alexia and agraphia in Chinese and in English. Chinese Medical Journal, 54:491-516.

Lynn, D. B. 1961.   Sex-role and parental identification. Mimeographed manuscript. University of Colorado School of Medicine.

McFie, J., and Zangwill, O. L. 1960.   Visual-constructive disabilities associated with lesions of the left cerebral hemisphere. Brain, 83:243-260.

McLaulin, J. C., and Schiffman, G. B. 1960. A study of the relationship between the California Test of Mental Maturity and the WISC test for retarded readers. Mimeographed manuscript. Board of Education, Baltimore County.

MacMahon, B., Pugh, T. F., and Ipsen, J. 1960. *Epidemiologic Methods.* Boston: Little, Brown.

Macmeeken, A. M. 1939. *Ocular Dominance in Relation to Developmental Aphasia.* London: University of London Press.

Maier, N. R. F., and Schneirla, T. C. 1935. *Principles of Animal Psychology.* New York: McGraw-Hill Book Co.

Malmquist, E. 1958. *Factors Related to Reading Disabilities in the First Grade.* Stockholm: Almqvist & Wiksell.

Margolin, J. B., Roman, M., and Harari, C. 1955. Reading disability in the delinquent child: a microcosm of psychosocial pathology. American Journal of Orthopsychiatry, 25:25-35.

Mark, H. J., and Hardy, W. G. 1958. Orienting reflex disturbances in central auditory or language handicapped children. Journal of Speech and Hearing Disorders, 23:237-242.

Maspes, P. E. 1948. Le syndrome expérimental chez l'homme de la section du splénium du corps calleux: alexie visuelle pure hémianopsique. Revue Neurologique, 80:100-113.

Meyer, A. 1950. Writings on aphasia. In *The Collected Papers of Adolf Meyer. Volume I: Neurology.* Baltimore: Johns Hopkins Press.

Miller, A. D., Margolin, J. B., and Yolles, S. F. 1957. Epidemiology of reading disabilities: some methodologic considerations and early findings. American Journal of Public Health, 47:1250-1256.

Milner, B. 1958. Psychological defects produced by temporal lobe excision. Research Publications of the Association for Research in Nervous and Mental Diseases, 36:244-257.

Money, J. 1961. Components of eroticism in man. II: The orgasm and genital somesthesia. Journal of Nervous and Mental Disease, 132:289-297.

Monroe, M. 1932. *Children Who Cannot Read.* Chicago: University of Chicago Press.

Mountcastle, V. B. (ed.) 1962. *Interhemispheric Relations and Cerebral Dominance.* Baltimore: Johns Hopkins Press. In press.

Naidoo, S. 1961. An investigation into some aspects of ambiguous handedness. M.A. Thesis. University of London.

Nielsen, J. M. 1946. Case 12. In *Agnosia, Apraxia, Aphasia.* New York: Paul B. Hoeber. P. 186.

Nunnally, J. C. Jr. 1959. *Tests and Measurements: Assessment and Prediction.* New York: McGraw-Hill Book Co.

Ombredane, A. 1937. Le méchanisme et la correction des difficultes de la lecture connues sous le nom de cécité verbale congénitale. Rapports de Psychiatrie Scolaire. Premier Congrès de Psychiatrie Infantile, Paris. Pp. 201-233.

Ombredane, A. 1951. *L'Aphasie et l'élaboration de la pensée explicite.* Paris: Presses Universitaires de France.

Orton, J. L. 1957. The Orton story. Bulletin of the Orton Society, 7:5-8.

Orton, S. T. 1934. Some studies in language function. Research Publications of the Association for Research in Nervous and Mental Disease, 13:614-633.

Orton, S. T. 1937. *Reading, Writing and Speech Problems in Children.* New York: W. W. Norton & Co.

O'Sullivan, M. A., and Pryles, C. V. 1962. Reading disability in children. Journal of Pediatrics, 60:369-375.

Paget, G. 1887. Notes on an exceptional case of aphasia. British Medical Journal, 2:1258-1259.

Panse, F., and Shimoyama, T. 1955. Zur Auswirkung aphasischer Störungen in Japanischen. II: Screib- und Lesestörungen. Archiv für Psychiatrie und Nervenkrankheiten, 193:139-145.

Parker School. 1957. The first seven years of the Gillingham reading program at Francis W. Parker School. Presented at the Gillingham Institute, The Francis W. Parker School, Chicago, Ill., January 26.

Pavlov, I. P. 1927. In *Conditioned Reflexes* (G. V. Anrep, ed.). Oxford: Oxford University Press.

Penfield, W., and Roberts, L. 1959. *Speech and Brain Mechanisms.* Princeton: Princeton University Press.

Perria, L., Rosadini, G., and Rossi, G. F. 1961. Determination of side of cerebral dominance with amobarbitol. Archives of Neurology, 4:173-181.

Piaget, J. 1955. *The Language and Thought of the Child.* New York: Meridian Press.

Piercy, M., Hécaen, H., and Ajuriaguerra, J. de. 1960. Constructional apraxia associated with unilateral cerebral lesions—left and right sided cases compared. Brain, 83:225-242.

Pitres, A. 1884. Considérations sur l'agraphie (agraphie motrice pure). Revue de Médecine, 4:855-873.

Prechtl, H. F. R., and Stemmer, J. C. 1959. Ein choreatiformes Syndrom bei Kindern. Wiener Medizinische Wochenschrift, 109:461-463.

Prechtl, H. F. R., and Stemmer, J. C. 1962. The choreiform syndrome in children. Developmental Medicine and Child Neurology, 4:119-127.

Rabinovitch, R. D. 1959. Reading and learning disabilities. In *American Handbook of Psychiatry* (S. Arieti, ed.). New York: Basic Books. Pp. 857-869.

Rabinovitch, R. D., Drew, A. L., De Jong, R. N., Ingram, W., and Withey, L. 1954. A research approach to reading retardation. Research Publications of the Association for Research in Nervous and Mental Disease, 34: 363-396.

Ranschburg, P. 1928. *Die Lese- und Schreibstörungen des Kindesalters.* Halle.

Renshaw, S. 1930. The errors of cutaneous localization and the effect of practice on the localizing movement in children and adults. Journal of Genetic Psychology, 38:223-238.

Renshaw, S. 1945. The visual perception and reproduction of forms by tachistoscopic methods. Journal of Psychology, 20:218-232.

Renshaw, S., Wherry, R. J., and Newlin, J. C. 1930. Cutaneous localization in congenitally blind versus seeing children and adults. Journal of Genetic Psychology, 38:239-248.

Riesen, A. H. 1958. Plasticity of behavior: psychological aspects. In *Biological and Biochemical Bases of Behavior* (H. F. Harlow and C. N. Woolsey, eds.). Madison: University of Wisconsin Press. Pp. 425-450.

Riesen, A. H. 1961. Studying perceptual development using the technique of sensory deprivation. Journal of Nervous and Mental Disease, 132:21-25.

Robinson, H. 1937. The study of disabilities in reading. Elementary School Journal, 38:1-14.

Robinson, H. M. 1946. *Why Pupils Fail in Reading.* Chicago: University of Chicago Press.

Rosen, G. 1958. *A History of Public Health.* New York: MD Publications.

Rosenberg, M. E. 1961. A brief look at the state of reading retardation. Laboratory report no. 1, Community Projects Section, Mental Health Study Center. Mimeographed manuscript.

Schiffman, G. B. 1957. How to organize a remedial reading program. In *Improving Reading in the Junior High,* Bulletin No. 10, United States Department of Health, Education and Welfare. Pp. 110-117.

Shepherd, E. M. 1956. Reading efficiency of 809 average school children. American Journal of Ophthalmology, 41:1029-1039.

Sherrington, C. S. 1951. *Man on His Nature.* Cambridge: Cambridge University Press.

Silver, A. A. 1952. Postural and righting responses in children. Journal of Pediatrics, 41:493-498.

Silver A. A., and Hagin, R. 1960. Specific reading disability: delineation of the syndrome and relationship to cerebral dominance. Comprehensive Psychiatry, 1:126-134.

Smith, D. E. P., and Carrigan, P. M. 1959. *The Nature of Reading Disability.* New York: Harcourt, Brace.

Smith, K. U. 1945. The role of the commissural systems of the cerebral cortex in the determination of handedness, eyedness and footedness in man. Journal of General Psychology, 32:39-79.

Sohval, A. R. 1961. Recent progress in human chromosome analysis and its relation to the sex chromatin. American Journal of Medicine, 31:397-441.

Sperry, R. W. 1961. Cerebral organization and behavior. Science, 133:1749-1757.

Statten, T. 1953. Behaviour patterns, reading disabilities and EEG findings. American Journal of Psychiatry, 110:205-206.

Subirana, A. 1958. The prognosis in aphasia in relation to the factor of cerebral dominance and handedness. · Brain, 81:415-425.

Sutherland, N. S. 1960. Visual discrimination of orientation by octopus: mirror images. British Journal of Psychology, 51:9-18.

Symonds, C. P. 1953. Aphasia. Journal of Neurology, Neurosurgery and Psychiatry. 16:1-6.

Taylor, J. (ed.) 1931. *The Selected Writings of John Hughlings Jackson.* London: Hodder & Stoughton.

Terman, L. M. 1926. *Genetic Studies of Genius.* Stanford: Stanford University Press.

Teuber, H.-L., Battersby, W. S., and Bender, M. B. 1960. *Visual Field Defects after Penetrating Missile Wounds of the Brain.* Cambridge, Mass.: Harvard University Press.

Thompson, L. 1956. Specific reading disability—Strephosymbolia. I: Diagnosis. Bulletin of the Orton Society, 6:3-9.

Thorndike, E. L., and Lorge, I. 1944. *The Teacher's Word Book of 30,000 Words.* New York: Teachers College, Columbia University.

Travis, L. E. 1931. *Speech Pathology.* New York: Appleton-Century.

Traxler, A. E., and Jungeblut, A. 1960. *Research in Reading During Another Four Years: Summary and Bibliography, July 1, 1953 to December 31, 1957.* New York: Educational Records Bureau.

Traxler, A. E., and Townsend, A. 1955. *Eight More Years of Research in Reading: Summary and Bibliography.* New York: Educational Records Bureau.

Trescher, J. H., and Ford, F. R. 1937. Colloid cyst of the third ventricle. Archives of Neurology and Psychiatry, 37:959-973.

Van Riper, C., and Butler, K. G. 1955. *Speech in the Elementary Classroom.* New York: Harper & Bros.

Vernon, M. D. 1957. *Backwardness in Reading.* Cambridge: Cambridge University Press.

Waggenheim, L. 1960. First memories of "accidents" and reading difficulties. American Journal of Orthopsychiatry, 30:191-195.

Walters, R. H., Van Loan, M., and Crofts, I. 1961. A study of reading disability. Journal of Consulting Psychology, 25:277-283.

Warrington, E., and Zangwill, O. L. 1957. A study of dyslexia. Journal of Neurology, Neurosurgery and Psychiatry, 20:208-215.

Wepman, J. M. 1958. *The Auditory Discrimination Test.* Chicago: Language Research Associates.

Wepman, J. M. 1960. Auditory discrimination, speech and reading. Elementary School Journal, 60:325-333.

Wepman, J. M. 1961. The interrelationship of hearing, speech and reading. The Reading Teacher, 14:245-247.

Wepman, J. M., Jones, L. V., Bock, R. D., and Van Pelt, D. 1960. Studies in aphasia: background and theoretical formulations. Journal of Speech and Hearing Disorders, 25:324-331.

Wernicke, C. 1874. *Die aphasische Symptomencomplex.* Breslau: Taschen.

Whorf, B. L. 1956. *Language, Thought and Reality.* Cambridge: Technology Press.

Zangwill, O. L. 1960. *Cerebral Dominance and Its Relation to Psychological Function.* Edinburgh: Oliver & Boyd.

Zangwill, O. L. 1961. Asymmetry of cerebral hemisphere function. In *Scientific Aspects of Neurology* (H. Garland, ed.). Edinburgh and London: Livingstone.

Addendum, second printing

Bauza, C. A. (ed.) 1962. *La Dislexia de Evolucion.* Montevideo, Garcia Morales-Mercant.

Franklin, A. W. (ed.) 1962. *Word-Blindness or Specific Developmental Dyslexia.* London, Pitman Medical Publishing Co.

Indexes

INDEX OF NAMES

214

INDEX OF SUBJECTS